The Complete Diabetes Cookbook for the Newly Diagnosed

Navigate Diabetes With Ease. Discover 1800 days of effortless, mouthwatering recipes that are low in sugar and carbs, including meal plans.

Table Of Content

Welcome to Your Deliciously Empowered Future: An Introduction to The Complete Diabetes Cookbook for the Newly Diagnosed

Being diagnosed with diabetes can bring a mix of emotions. It's like discovering something new about your body—something you might not have expected. I'm here to tell you that it's okay if you feel a bit surprised, confused, or even a little worried. Many people share those feelings when they first hear the news. The important thing to know is that you're not alone, and there's a wealth of support and information available to help you navigate this new chapter in your life. Think of being diagnosed with diabetes as embarking on a journey—a journey where you become the captain of your own ship. Yes, there might be challenges along the way, but there's also an opportunity for growth, learning, and discovering how resilient and capable you truly are.

Understanding diabetes is a crucial step in this journey. It's not just a condition; it's a part of your life that requires paying more attention and care to what you eat and drink. Diabetes affects how your body handles a sugar called glucose, which comes from the food you eat. Normally, your body produces a hormone called insulin to help manage this glucose, but in diabetes, this process doesn't work as smoothly as it should. The good news is that by learning about diabetes, you gain the power to make informed choices about your health. It's like having a roadmap or a blueprint that helps you go through the twists and turns of managing your blood sugar levels. And that's where our cookbook comes in—as your trusted guide, helping you navigate the cooking aspects of this journey.

Let's talk about food. Food is not just fuel for your body; it's an important part of your life, culture, and enjoyment. The idea is not to take away your favorites but to find a balance that keeps you feeling good. Our cookbook is designed to make this balance not only achievable but also delicious. Picture this: your meals become moments of celebration, a time to savor both the flavors and the nourishment your body needs. Breakfast, lunch, and dinner transform into opportunities to explore new recipes, try different ingredients, and discover the joy of preparing meals that love you back.

Snacks, too, play a vital role in this journey. They're not just fillers but delightful interludes between meals. With a bit of creativity, you can turn snack time into a delightful experience, filled with treats that not only satisfy but also keep your blood sugar levels in check. Now, I know change can feel overwhelming, but let me assure you—you don't have to do it all at once. This journey is about progress, not perfection. Take small, manageable steps. Maybe start by experimenting with a new recipe or gradually incorporating more vegetables into your meals. As these small changes become habits, you'll find that managing diabetes becomes a natural part of your routine.

And guess what? You're not alone on this journey. Your friends, family, and healthcare practioners are like your trusted companions, ready to support and encourage you. Share your concerns, celebrate your victories, and let them be part of this adventure with you.

Exercising your body is another important part of managing diabetes. But don't worry, you don't need to run a marathon. It can be as simple as taking a stroll in the neighborhood, doing a little dance in your living room, or trying out a gentle yoga routine. Find activities you enjoy, and let them be moments of joy and self-care.

Stress management is also a key player in this game. Life can be hectic, and stress might try to sneak in. But you have the power to keep it in check. Whether it's through deep breaths, finding a quiet moment, or pursuing a hobby you love, taking time for yourself is a crucial part of your well-being.

Here you are – at the beginning of your diabetes journey. It's a journey of self-discovery, resilience, and embracing a new way of living. Think of it as an adventure, where each day brings new opportunities to learn, grow, and savor the richness of life.

So, as you turn the pages of your story, let our cookbook be a companion, guiding you through the culinary delights of this journey. From appetizers to desserts, each recipe is a step towards a healthier and happier you. Your diabetes journey is not a sprint; it's a marathon, and you have the strength, knowledge, and support to make it a fulfilling and joyful one. So, let's lace up those shoes, gather our ingredients, and step into this adventure together!

Understanding the Basics: Diabetes and Food's Impact on Blood Sugar

A diagnosis of diabetes can feel like stepping into uncharted territory. But fear not, for knowledge is your map, and we're here to guide you through the basics of this condition and how your food choices influence your blood sugar levels.

What is Diabetes?

Imagine your body as a power plant. Glucose, a type of sugar from food, acts as the fuel, and insulin, a hormone produced by your pancreas, works like the key that unlocks the cells, allowing glucose to enter and provide energy. In diabetes, this system malfunctions.

Blood Sugar Rollercoaster:
In both types, the result is the same: glucose builds up in your bloodstream instead of entering your cells, causing high blood sugar levels (hyperglycemia). This is like having too much fuel sitting in the tank, unused. Over time, uncontrolled high blood sugar can damage your eyes, nerves, kidneys, and heart.

Food and the Blood Sugar Spike:
Now, let's talk food. When you eat, carbohydrates (found in sugars, starches, and grains) are broken down into glucose, causing your blood sugar to rise. Think of this as pouring more fuel into the tank.

The Glycemic Index (GI):
This handy tool ranks foods based on their blood sugar-raising effect. Low-GI foods (like vegetables and beans) cause gradual rises, while high-GI foods (like white bread and sugary drinks) spike blood sugar quickly. Choosing low-GI foods can help you manage your diabetes effectively.

Fueling Your Body Wisely:
Remember, managing diabetes isn't about deprivation; it's about making informed choices. Focus on:
- Whole grains: Opt for brown rice, quinoa, oats, and whole-wheat bread for sustainable energy and fiber.
- Lean protein: Chicken, fish, beans, lentils, and tofu keep you feeling full and regulate blood sugar.
- Healthy fats: Avocados, nuts, seeds, and olive oil provide essential fats and satiety. Choose monounsaturated and polyunsaturated fats over saturated and trans fats.
- Low-glycemic fruits and vegetables: Fill your plate with berries, apples, leafy greens, broccoli, and cauliflower for vitamins, minerals, and sustained energy.

- Limiting sugary drinks and processed foods: These contribute to spikes in blood sugar and offer little nutritional value.

By understanding the basics of diabetes and how food affects your blood sugar levels, you can make informed choices to manage your health effectively. Remember, you're not alone on this journey. Explore this book for delicious recipes, helpful tips, and inspiring stories to empower you every step of the way.

Kitchen Must-Haves for Managing Diabetes

Essential Appliances:
- Spiralizer: Ditch high-carb pasta for spiralized zucchini, butternut squash, or potatoes. It's a fun and low-glycemic way to enjoy your favorite pasta dishes.
- Blender/Food Processor: Whip up healthy smoothies, sauces, dips, and veggie dressings packed with nutrients.
- Slow Cooker: Set it and forget it! Ideal for preparing slow-cooked meats, soups, and stews that are bursting with flavor and perfect for meal prepping.
- Air Fryer: This healthier alternative to deep frying allows you to enjoy crispy veggies, fish, and even tofu without the guilt.
- Instant Pot: A multi-cooker that can steam, pressure cook, slow cook, and more. Saves time and simplifies preparation for various diabetic-friendly meals.

Items For Your Pantry:
- Whole Grains: Stock up on quinoa, brown rice, barley, and whole-wheat bread for satisfying fiber and slow-releasing carbs.
- Nuts and Seeds: Almonds, walnuts, chia seeds, and flaxseeds are excellent sources of healthy fats, protein, and fiber. Sprinkle them on salads, yogurt, or trail mix.
- Spices and Herbs: Experiment with cinnamon, turmeric, ginger, cumin, coriander, and fresh herbs like basil, parsley, and cilantro. They add flavor without adding sugar or sodium.
- Low-Sodium Canned Beans and Lentils: A protein and fiber powerhouse, perfect for adding to salads, soups, and dips. Choose BPA-free options.
- Vinegar and Olive Oil: Healthy alternatives to sugary sauces and dressings. Drizzle on salads or use for marinades.
- Low-Sugar Canned Fruits and Vegetables: Keep options like diced tomatoes, artichoke hearts, and unsweetened beans on hand for quick and healthy additions to meals.

Fridge Essentials:
- Non-starchy Vegetables: Load up on leafy greens, broccoli, cauliflower, peppers, carrots, and zucchini. They're low in carbs and packed with vitamins and minerals.
- Low-Fat Yogurt and Cheese: Great sources of protein and calcium. Choose plain yogurt and add your own berries or nuts for sweetness.
- Lean Protein: Stock up on fish, chicken, turkey, and eggs for healthy fats and protein to keep you feeling full and satisfied.
- Healthy Fats: Avocado, olives, and nut butters provide healthy fats and fiber, aiding in satiety and blood sugar control.

Bonus Tools:
- Portion Control Containers: Pre-portioned containers help with mindful eating and carb counting.
- Kitchen Scale: Precise measurement of ingredients is key for accurate carb counting.
- Reusable Food Storage Bags and Containers: Reduce waste and keep food fresh for meal prepping and on-the-go snacks.

Remember:
- Make it colorful! A variety of fruits and vegetables ensures you're getting a diverse range of vitamins and minerals.
- Don't forget the water! Staying hydrated is crucial for overall health and can also help prevent cravings.
- Plan your meals: Planning ahead takes away the stress of last-minute decisions that might lead to unhealthy choices.
- Get creative! Experiment with different spices, herbs, and cooking methods to keep things interesting.

Make it a family affair! Get your family involved in choosing and preparing healthy meals.

By equipping your kitchen with these essentials, you'll be well on your way to creating a diabetes-friendly haven where deliciousness meets health. Remember, managing diabetes is a journey, and your kitchen is your constant companion. Make it a source of inspiration, creativity, and support, and you'll find yourself not just managing your blood sugar, but thriving in the kitchen and beyond.

Weekly Meal Plans Just For You

Day 1:
Breakfast:
- Scrambled eggs with spinach and tomatoes
- Whole grain toast

Lunch:
- Grilled chicken salad with mixed greens, cherry tomatoes, cucumber, and vinaigrette dressing

Dinner:
- Baked salmon with quinoa
- Steamed broccoli and carrots

Snack:
- Greek yogurt with berries

Day 2:
Breakfast:
- Overnight oats with almond milk, chia seeds, and sliced bananas

Lunch:
- Turkey and avocado wrap with whole grain tortilla

Dinner:
- Stir-fried tofu with brown rice and mixed vegetables

Snack:
- Handful of mixed nuts

Day 3:
Breakfast:
- Smoothie with spinach, banana, almond milk, and protein powder

Lunch:
- Quinoa salad with black beans, corn, cherry tomatoes, and lime dressing

Dinner:
- Grilled shrimp with sweet potato wedges
- Asparagus spears

Snack:
- Apple slices with peanut butter

Day 4:
Breakfast:
- Whole grain pancakes with maple syrup and a side of berries

Lunch:
- Lentil soup with a side of whole grain bread

Dinner:
- Grilled chicken breast with roasted Brussels sprouts and quinoa

Snack:
- Hummus with carrot and cucumber sticks

Day 5:
Breakfast:
- Greek yogurt parfait with granola and mixed berries

Lunch:
- Caprese salad with mozzarella, tomatoes, and basil drizzled with balsamic glaze

Dinner:
- Baked cod with lemon and herbs
- Brown rice and steamed green beans

Snack:
- Cottage cheese with pineapple chunks

Day 6:
Breakfast:
- Avocado toast with poached eggs

Lunch:
- Chickpea salad with feta cheese, cherry tomatoes, and olives

Dinner:
- Beef stir-fry with broccoli and brown rice

Snack:
- Banana with almond butter

Day 7:
Breakfast:
- Omelette with mushrooms, onions, and bell peppers
- Whole grain toast

Lunch:
- Turkey and vegetable kebabs with quinoa

Dinner:
- Baked chicken thighs with sweet potato mash and green beans

Snack:

- Mixed fruit bowl (strawberries, blueberries, and kiwi)

Day 8:
Breakfast:
- Smoothie bowl with mixed berries, banana, granola, and a dollop of Greek yogurt

Lunch:
- Spinach and feta stuffed chicken breast with a side of quinoa

Dinner:
- Baked cod with a mango salsa topping
- Steamed asparagus and brown rice

Snack:
- Handful of cherry tomatoes with mozzarella cheese

Day 9:
Breakfast:
- Scrambled tofu with sautéed mushrooms and whole grain toast

Lunch:
- Turkey and vegetable stir-fry with broccoli and snow peas, served with brown rice

Dinner:
- Grilled salmon with a dill and lemon marinade
- Quinoa and roasted sweet potato cubes

Snack:
- Carrot and cucumber slices with tzatziki dip

Day 10:
Breakfast:
- Chia seed pudding with almond milk, topped with sliced strawberries and a drizzle of honey

Lunch:
- Black bean and vegetable wrap with salsa and avocado

Dinner:
- Stir-fried shrimp with a mix of colorful bell peppers and cauliflower rice

Snack:
- Mixed nuts and dried fruit

Day 11:
Breakfast:
- Whole grain waffles with fresh fruit (such as blueberries and raspberries) and a dollop of whipped cream

Lunch:
- Quinoa and chickpea salad with diced cucumber, cherry tomatoes, and a lemon vinaigrette

Dinner:
- Grilled chicken thighs with rosemary and garlic
- Mashed sweet potatoes and steamed broccoli

Snack:
- Apple slices with cheese slices

Day 12:

Breakfast:
- Veggie omelette with tomatoes, bell peppers, onions, and a sprinkle of cheese

Lunch:
- Lentil and vegetable curry with brown rice

Dinner:
- Baked tilapia with a mango and avocado salsa
- Quinoa and sautéed green beans

Snack:
- Greek yogurt with a drizzle of honey

Day 13:

Breakfast:
- Banana and almond butter smoothie with a handful of spinach

Lunch:
- Caprese quinoa bowl with cherry tomatoes, fresh mozzarella, and basil

Dinner:
- Turkey meatballs with marinara sauce over whole grain spaghetti
- Roasted Brussels sprouts

Snack:
- Trail mix with nuts and dried fruit

Day 14:

Breakfast:
- Avocado and smoked salmon on whole grain toast

Lunch:
- Chickpea and vegetable curry with quinoa

Dinner:
- Beef and vegetable kebabs with a side of wild rice

Snack:
- Cottage cheese with pineapple chunks

Day 15
Breakfast;
- Baked Apple Oatmeal with berries and walnuts

Lunch;
- Greek Chicken Souvlaki Salad with grilled chicken, mixed greens, feta cheese, and olives

Dinner;
- Grilled Lemon Herb Salmon with roasted Brussels sprouts and quinoa

Snacks;
- Cucumber Hummus Bites: Sliced cucumber with hummus for a refreshing and protein-packed snack.

Day 16
Breakfast;
- Chia Seed Pudding with almond milk, chia seeds, and berries

Lunch;
- Cauliflower Fried Rice with shrimp and vegetables

Dinner;
- Grilled shrimp with sweet potato wedges

Snacks;
- Avocado and Tomato Salsa Cups: Mini bell peppers filled with chopped avocado and tomato salsa for a satisfying bite.

Day 17
Breakfast:
- Almond Flour Banana Muffins with Greek yogurt and sliced avocado

Lunch:
- Mediterranean Quinoa Salad with quinoa, chickpeas, cucumber, tomatoes, and feta cheese

Dinner:
- Lemon Garlic Herb Grilled Chicken with roasted asparagus and mashed cauliflower

Snacks:
- Cheese and Veggie Kabobs: Cherry tomatoes, mozzarella cheese, and cucumber skewers drizzled with balsamic glaze.

Day 18
Breakfast:

- Mango and Lime Overnight Oats with chopped nuts and seeds

Lunch:

- Black Bean and Corn Salad with grilled chicken, black beans, corn, and avocado

Dinner:

- Teriyaki Tofu Stir-Fry with tofu, vegetables, and teriyaki sauce

Snacks:

- Spiced Roasted Chickpeas: A crunchy and flavorful snack with roasted chickpeas seasoned with herbs and spices.

Day 19

Breakfast:

- Spinach and Feta Breakfast Wrap with a whole-wheat tortilla

Lunch:

- Cabbage and Turkey Sauté with cabbage, ground turkey, bell peppers, and spices

Dinner:

- Indian-Spiced Lentil Curry with lentils, vegetables, and spices

Snacks:

- Almond Butter-Stuffed Dates: Medjool dates stuffed with almond butter for a natural energy boost.

Day 20

Breakfast:

- Peanut Butter and Banana Toast on whole-wheat bread with sliced almonds

Lunch:

- Spinach and Feta Stuffed Chicken Breast with spinach, feta, and quinoa

Dinner:

- Grilled Lemon Herb Salmon with roasted broccoli and brown rice

Snacks:

- Caprese Salad Skewers: Cherry tomatoes, fresh mozzarella, and basil leaves on skewers for a mini caprese salad.

Day 21

Breakfast:

- Veggie and Cheese Omelette Wrap with bell peppers, spinach, and low-fat cheese

Lunch:

- Lentil and Vegetable Curry with lentils, vegetables, and spices

Dinner:

- Roasted Vegetable and Chickpea Salad with roasted vegetables, chickpeas, and herbs

Snacks:

- Guacamole Deviled Eggs: Hard-boiled eggs filled with guacamole for a protein-rich snack.

Day 22

Breakfast:
- Turkey and Vegetable Skillet with quinoa, diced turkey, vegetables, and spices

Lunch:
- Veggies and Hummus Wrap with hummus, vegetables, and a whole-wheat tortilla

Dinner:
- Turkey and Vegetable Lettuce Wraps with ground turkey, vegetables, and lettuce wraps

Snacks;
- Cottage Cheese and Pineapple Cups: Cottage cheese mixed with chopped pineapple for a sweet and creamy snack.

Day 23

Breakfast;
- Cottage Cheese Pancakes topped with fruit and chia seeds

Lunch;
- Stuffed Portobello Mushrooms with quinoa, vegetables, and herbs

Dinner;
- Spaghetti Squash Primavera with spaghetti squash, vegetables, and herbs

Snacks;
- Turmeric Roasted Almonds: A healthy and flavorful snack with almonds roasted in turmeric and herbs.

Day 24

Breakfast;
- Salmon and Dill Frittata with smoked salmon, eggs, and herbs

Lunch;
- Turkey and Vegetable Skillet with quinoa, diced turkey, vegetables, and spices

Dinner;
- Zucchini Noodles with Pesto and Cherry Tomatoes with grilled chicken

Snack;
- Seaweed and Smoked Salmon Rolls: Nori seaweed sheets wrapped around smoked salmon for a savory and low-carb snack.

Day 25

Breakfast;
- Protein-Packed Smoothie Bowl with Greek yogurt, protein powder, berries, and granola

Lunch;

- Cucumber and Avocado Gazpacho with cucumber, avocado, tomato, and herbs

Dinner;

- Cajun Shrimp and Sausage Skillet with shrimp, sausage, vegetables, and spices

Snacks;

- Berries and Ricotta Toast: Whole-wheat toast topped with ricotta cheese and fresh berries for a light and delicious snack.

Day 26

Breakfast;

- Coconut Flour Waffles with sugar-free syrup and berries

Lunch;

- Pesto Zoodle Bowl with zucchini noodles, pesto, and grilled chicken

Dinner;

- Balsamic Glazed Turkey Meatballs with roasted vegetables and brown rice

Snacks;

- Zucchini Chips with Parmesan: Baked zucchini slices sprinkled with parmesan cheese for a crispy and healthy snack.

Day 27

Breakfast;

- Greek Yogurt Parfait with fruit, nuts, and chia seeds

Lunch;

- Greek Chicken Souvlaki Salad with grilled chicken, mixed greens, feta cheese, and olives

Dinner;

- Greek Chicken Souvlaki Bowl with grilled chicken, quinoa, tzatziki sauce, and vegetables

Snacks;

- Edamame and Sea Salt Pods: A good source of fiber and protein, edamame pods are a satisfying snack.

Day 28

Breakfast;

- Egg and Vegetable Muffin Cups with spinach, tomatoes, and eggs

Lunch;

- Salmon and Avocado Wrap with whole-wheat tortilla, smoked salmon, and avocado

Dinner;

- Stuffed Bell Peppers with Quinoa and Black Beans with bell peppers, quinoa, black beans, and vegetables

Snacks;

- Mango Chili Lime Salsa: Made with fresh mango, jalapeño, and lime, this salsa can be enjoyed with chips or vegetables.

Day 29
Breakfast;
- Mushroom and Spinach Egg Cups with herbs and spices

Lunch;
- Roasted Vegetable and Chickpea Salad with roasted vegetables, chickpeas, and herbs

Dinner;
- Butter Herb Roasted Vegetables with Chicken with roasted vegetables and grilled chicken

Snacks;
- Walnut-Stuffed Celery: Celery sticks filled with cream cheese and chopped walnuts for a crunchy and creamy snack.

Day 30
Breakfast;
- Breakfast Burrito Bowl with scrambled eggs, black beans, avocado, and salsa

Lunch;
- Tuna Salad Lettuce Wraps with tuna salad, lettuce wraps, and sliced vegetables

Dinner
- Baked Cod with Mediterranean Salsa with baked cod, Mediterranean salsa, and brown rice

Snacks;
- Chocolate-Dipped Strawberries: Fresh strawberries dipped in dark chocolate for a satisfying sweet treat.

The thirty-day meal plan provided above is designed to offer a diverse and balanced approach to nutrition. It serves as a flexible template that can be easily adjusted to accommodate your individual preferences, dietary requirements, and lifestyle. Feel free to interchange meals between days, modify portion sizes, or incorporate alternative ingredients based on your tastes and nutritional goals.

Weekly Grocery Shopping List

Week 1:

Proteins:
- Skinless chicken breast
- Salmon fillets
- Lean ground turkey
- Eggs

Vegetables:
- Broccoli
- Spinach
- Bell peppers
- Zucchini
- Tomatoes

Fruits:
- Berries (blueberries, strawberries)
- Avocado
- Lemons

Whole Grains:
- Quinoa
- Brown rice
- Whole grain oats

Dairy:
- Greek yogurt (unsweetened)
- Low-fat cheese

Legumes:
- Black beans
- Chickpeas

Nuts and Seeds:
- Almonds
- Chia seeds
- Flaxseeds

Condiments and Sauces:
- Olive oil
- Balsamic vinegar
- Dijon mustard
- Low-sodium soy sauce

Others:
- Garlic
- Low-sodium vegetable broth
- Herbs and spices (rosemary, thyme, cumin, paprika)

Week 2:

Proteins:
- Tofu
- Shrimp
- Ground chicken
- Cottage cheese

Vegetables:
- Asparagus
- Brussels sprouts
- Cauliflower
- Cucumbers

Fruits:
- Oranges
- Apples
- Pears

Whole Grains:
- Barley
- Whole wheat pasta

Dairy:
- Unsweetened almond milk

Legumes:
- Lentils

Nuts and Seeds:
- Walnuts
- Sunflower seeds

Condiments and Sauces
- Tomato sauce (low-sugar)
- Apple cider vinegar

Others:
- Ginger
- Low-sodium chicken broth

Week 3:

Proteins:
- Pork loin
- Turkey bacon
- Eggs

Vegetables:
- Kale
- Eggplant
- Green beans
- Radishes

Fruits:
- Grapefruit
- Kiwi

Whole Grains:
- Bulgur
- Farro

Dairy:
- Low-fat plain yogurt

Legumes:
- Pinto beans

Nuts and Seeds:
- Pecans
- Pumpkin seeds

Condiments and Sauces:
- Salsa (no added sugar)
- Hot sauce

Others:
- Low-sodium beef broth
- Fresh herbs (cilantro, parsley)

Week 4:
Proteins:
- Lean beef sirloin
- Chicken thighs
- Smoked salmon
- Eggs

Vegetables:
- Cabbage
- Bell peppers
- Cherry tomatoes
- Mushrooms

Fruits:
- Mango
- Pineapple

Whole Grains:
- Millet
- Buckwheat

Dairy:
- Low-fat milk

Legumes:
- Edamame

Nuts and Seeds:
- Cashews
- Sesame seeds

Condiments and Sauces:
- Low-fat salad dressing
- Low-sodium teriyaki sauce

Others:
- Green onions
- Low-sodium vegetable juice

Make sure to adjust the amounts according to what works for you, and always ensure to look at the labels for any extra sugars and salt. Fresh veggies are good, but don't sleep on frozen ones—they're easy and still super healthy.

Breakfasts to Start Your Day Right

Veggie and Cheese Omelette Wrap

Ingredients:

- 2 large eggs
- 1/4 cup bell peppers (mixed colors), diced
- 1/4 cup cherry tomatoes, halved
- 1/4 cup spinach, chopped
- 2 tablespoons red onion, finely chopped
- 1/4 cup shredded cheese (cheddar or your favorite blend)
- Salt and pepper to taste
- 1 tablespoon olive oil

Servings:

This recipe makes one generously sized Veggie and Cheese Omelette Wrap.

Instructions:

- Prepare the Vegetables:Dice the bell peppers, halve the cherry tomatoes, chop the spinach, and finely chop the red onion.
- Whisk the Eggs:In a bowl, whisk the two large eggs until well combined. Season with salt and pepper to taste.
- Sauté the Vegetables:Heat olive oil in a non-stick skillet over medium heat. Add the bell peppers, cherry tomatoes, spinach, and red onion. Sauté until the vegetables are tender but still vibrant.
- Pour in the Eggs:Pour the whisked eggs over the sautéed vegetables, ensuring an even distribution. Allow the eggs to set at the edges.
- Add the Cheese:Sprinkle the shredded cheese evenly over one half of the omelette.
- Fold and Cook:Carefully fold the omelette in half, covering the cheese. Press gently with a spatula and let it cook for another minute until the cheese melts and the eggs are fully set.
- Serve Warm:Slide the Veggie and Cheese Omelette onto a plate and serve immediately.
- Optional: Wrap it Up!For an extra touch, serve the omelette inside a whole-grain or low-carb wrap for a portable and convenient meal.

Enjoy your Veggie and Cheese Omelette Wrap

Greek Yogurt Parfait

Ingredients:

- 1 cup Greek yogurt (unsweetened)
- 1/2 cup granola (choose a low-sugar or homemade option)
- 1/2 cup mixed berries (strawberries, blueberries, raspberries)

- 1 tablespoon honey (optional, for drizzling)
- 1 tablespoon chopped nuts (almonds, walnuts, or pistachios)
- Servings: 1

Instructions:
- Lay the Base:In a serving glass or bowl, spoon a layer of Greek yogurt at the bottom. This will be the base of your parfait.
- Add Granola:Sprinkle a layer of granola over the Greek yogurt. Ensure an even distribution for a satisfying crunch in every bite.
- Introduce the Berries:Place a layer of mixed berries over the granola. Feel free to mix and match or create a pattern for an aesthetically pleasing presentation.
- Repeat Layers:Repeat the layers of Greek yogurt, granola, and berries until you reach the top of the glass or bowl. This creates a visually appealing and deliciously textured parfait.
- Drizzle with Honey (Optional):If you desire a touch of sweetness, drizzle honey over the top of your parfait. Adjust the quantity based on your personal preference.
- Garnish with Chopped Nuts:Sprinkle chopped nuts over the parfait for added texture and a nutrient boost. Choose your favorite nuts or a mix for variety.
- Serve Immediately:Your Greek Yogurt Parfait is ready to be enjoyed! Serve it immediately to savor the contrast of creamy yogurt, crunchy granola, sweet berries, and nutty goodness.
- Customize (Optional):Feel free to customize your parfait with additional toppings such as shredded coconut, chia seeds, or a sprinkle of cinnamon for extra flavor.

Note:This recipe is versatile, allowing you to adjust ingredient quantities based on personal preferences and dietary requirements.

Chia Seed Pudding

Ingredients:
- 1/4 cup chia seeds
- 1 cup almond milk (or any preferred milk)
- 1-2 tablespoons sweetener of choice (such as honey, maple syrup, or stevia)
- 1/2 teaspoon vanilla extract
- Fresh berries or sliced fruits for topping (optional)
- Nuts or seeds for garnish (optional)

Servings: 2

Instructions:
- In a bowl, combine the chia seeds, almond milk, sweetener, and vanilla extract. Whisk well to ensure the chia seeds are evenly distributed.
- Cover the bowl and refrigerate the mixture for at least 4 hours or preferably overnight. This allows the chia seeds to absorb the liquid and create a pudding-like consistency.

- After the initial setting time, give the chia seed mixture a good stir. If it's too thick for your liking, you can add a bit more milk to achieve your desired consistency.
- Spoon the chia seed pudding into serving glasses or bowls.
- Garnish with fresh berries, sliced fruits, nuts, or seeds for added texture and flavor.
- Your Chia Seed Pudding is now ready to be enjoyed! Serve it as a nutritious breakfast, a satisfying snack, or a guilt-free dessert.

Avocado and Smoked Salmon Toast

Ingredients:
- 2 slices of whole-grain or low-carb bread
- 1 ripe avocado
- 100g smoked salmon
- Fresh dill, for garnish
- Lemon wedges, for serving
- Salt and pepper, to taste

Servings: 2

Instructions:
- Toast the slices of bread to your preferred level of crispiness. Use whole-grain or low-carb bread for a healthier option.
- While the bread is toasting, cut the ripe avocado in half, remove the pit, and scoop the flesh into a bowl. Mash the avocado with a fork until it reaches your desired consistency.
- Season the mashed avocado with a pinch of salt and pepper. Mix well to ensure the seasoning is evenly distributed.
- Spread the seasoned mashed avocado evenly over the toasted bread slices.
- Place slices of smoked salmon on top of the mashed avocado. Ensure an even distribution to cover the entire surface of the toast.
- Finely chop fresh dill and sprinkle it over the smoked salmon. The dill adds a burst of freshness and complements the flavors.
- Serve the avocado and smoked salmon toast with lemon wedges on the side. Squeezing fresh lemon juice over the toast adds a zesty kick.
- Optional:Customize your toast by adding extras like a poached egg, cherry tomatoes, or red onion slices for additional flavor and texture.
- Your Avocado and Smoked Salmon Toast is ready to be enjoyed! This dish is perfect for breakfast, brunch, or a light and satisfying lunch.

Quinoa Breakfast Bowl

Ingredients:
- 1 cup quinoa
- 2 cups water

- 1 cup almond milk (or any preferred milk)
- 1 tablespoon honey or maple syrup (optional)
- 1 teaspoon vanilla extract
- 1/2 teaspoon cinnamon
- Fresh fruits (berries, sliced banana, or your choice)
- Nuts and seeds (almonds, chia seeds, pumpkin seeds)
- Greek yogurt or dairy-free alternative
- Drizzle of honey (optional)

Servings: 2

Instructions:

Rinse Quinoa:

- Rinse the quinoa under cold water to remove any bitterness.

Cook Quinoa:

- In a medium saucepan, combine the rinsed quinoa and water.
- Bring to a boil, then reduce the heat to low, cover, and simmer for 15 minutes or until the quinoa is cooked and water is absorbed.
- Fluff the quinoa with a fork.

Prepare Quinoa Base:

- In a separate saucepan, warm the almond milk over medium heat. Add the cooked quinoa to the almond milk.
- Stir in honey or maple syrup (if using), vanilla extract, and cinnamon.
- Cook for an additional 2-3 minutes until the mixture is heated through and well combined.

Assemble Breakfast Bowls:

- Divide the quinoa mixture into two bowls.

Add Toppings:

- Top each bowl with a generous amount of fresh fruits, nuts, seeds, and a dollop of Greek yogurt or dairy-free alternative.

Drizzle with Honey (Optional):

- For added sweetness, drizzle a bit of honey over the top.

Serve and Enjoy:

- Your Quinoa Breakfast Bowl is now ready to be served.
- Mix the ingredients together or enjoy the toppings separately for a delightful and nutritious breakfast.

Sweet Potato Hash with Turkey Sausage

Ingredients:

- 2 medium-sized sweet potatoes, peeled and diced
- 1 pound turkey sausage, casings removed

- 1 onion, finely chopped
- 1 bell pepper, diced
- 2 cloves garlic, minced
- 2 tablespoons olive oil
- 1 teaspoon smoked paprika
- 1/2 teaspoon dried thyme
- Salt and pepper to taste
- Fresh parsley for garnish (optional)

Servings: 4

Instructions:

Prepare Ingredients:
- Peel and dice the sweet potatoes into small, uniform cubes.
- Remove the casings from the turkey sausage.

Sauté Vegetables:
- In a large skillet, heat the olive oil over medium heat.
- Add the chopped onion and bell pepper, sautéing until softened, about 3-4 minutes.
- Stir in the minced garlic and cook for an additional 1-2 minutes until fragrant.

Cook Turkey Sausage:
- Add the turkey sausage to the skillet, breaking it into crumbles with a spatula.
- Cook until the turkey is browned and cooked through, ensuring it is evenly distributed with the vegetables.

Add Sweet Potatoes and Season:
- Incorporate the diced sweet potatoes into the skillet, mixing well with the sausage and vegetables.
- Season the mixture with smoked paprika, dried thyme, salt, and pepper. Adjust the seasoning to taste.

Cover and Cook:
- Cover the skillet and let the sweet potato hash cook over medium heat for about 15-20 minutes, stirring occasionally. Ensure the sweet potatoes are tender but not mushy.

Finish and Garnish:
- Once the sweet potatoes are cooked, uncover the skillet and let the hash cook for an additional 5 minutes, allowing the edges to crisp up slightly.
- Garnish with fresh parsley if desired.

Serve:
- Divide the sweet potato hash into four servings and plate it hot.
- This dish can be enjoyed on its own or paired with a fried or poached egg for added protein and richness.

Egg and Vegetable Muffin Cups

Ingredients:
- 6 large eggs
- 1 cup diced bell peppers (mix of red, yellow, and green)
- 1/2 cup diced red onion
- 1 cup chopped spinach leaves
- 1/2 cup grated cheddar cheese
- Salt and pepper to taste
- Cooking spray or butter for greasing muffin tin

Servings: 6 muffin cups

Instructions:
- Preheat your oven to 375°F (190°C).
- Grease a 6-cup muffin tin with cooking spray or butter to prevent sticking.
- Crack the eggs into a bowl and whisk them until well-beaten. Season with salt and pepper to taste.
- In a separate bowl, combine diced bell peppers, red onion, and chopped spinach.
- Pour the beaten eggs over the vegetable mixture. Add grated cheddar cheese and gently mix until ingredients are evenly distributed.
- Spoon the egg and vegetable mixture into each muffin cup, filling them about two-thirds full.
- Place the muffin tin in the preheated oven and bake for 20-25 minutes or until the tops are golden brown, and the eggs are set.
- To ensure the muffin cups are cooked through, insert a toothpick into the center of one; it should come out clean when they are done.
- Allow the muffin cups to cool in the tin for a few minutes before transferring them to a wire rack. Serve warm.

Spinach and Feta Breakfast Wrap

Ingredients:
- 1 large whole-grain or low-carb tortilla
- 2 large eggs
- 1 cup fresh spinach leaves, washed and patted dry
- 1/4 cup crumbled feta cheese
- Salt and pepper to taste
- Olive oil or cooking spray for the pan

Servings:1 serving

Instructions:

Preparation:

- Heat a non-stick skillet over medium heat.
- While the skillet is heating, whisk the eggs in a bowl and season with salt and pepper to taste.

Cooking the Eggs:

- Add a small amount of olive oil or cooking spray to the skillet.
- Pour the whisked eggs into the skillet, stirring gently with a spatula.
- Cook the eggs until they are just set but still moist, about 2-3 minutes.

Adding Spinach:

- Add the fresh spinach leaves to the skillet with the cooked eggs.
- Stir the spinach into the eggs, allowing it to wilt slightly. This should take an additional 1-2 minutes.

Creating the Wrap:

- Place the tortilla on a flat surface.
- Spoon the cooked eggs and spinach mixture onto the center of the tortilla.

Adding Feta:

- Sprinkle the crumbled feta cheese evenly over the egg and spinach mixture.

Wrapping It Up:

- Fold the sides of the tortilla toward the center, and then roll it up from the bottom, creating a wrap.

Final Touch:

- Place the wrapped breakfast in the skillet for an additional minute, seam side down, to seal the wrap and lightly toast the tortilla.

Serve:

- Transfer the spinach and feta breakfast wrap to a plate and serve immediately.

Cottage Cheese Pancakes

Ingredients:

- 1 cup cottage cheese
- 2 large eggs
- 1/4 cup almond flour
- 1/2 teaspoon baking powder
- 1 tablespoon sweetener of choice (optional)
- 1 teaspoon vanilla extract
- Butter or oil for cooking

Servings: 2-3 servings (makes approximately 6 pancakes)

Instructions:

Prepare the Batter:

- In a blender or food processor, combine the cottage cheese, eggs, almond flour, baking powder, sweetener (if using), and vanilla extract.
- Blend until the mixture is smooth and well combined.

Let the Batter Rest:

- Allow the batter to rest for a few minutes. This helps the almond flour absorb moisture and contributes to fluffier pancakes.

Preheat the Pan:

- Heat a non-stick skillet or griddle over medium heat. Add a small amount of butter or oil to coat the surface.

Cooking the Pancakes:

- Pour 1/4 cup portions of the batter onto the heated skillet. Spread the batter slightly to form even circles.

Flip and Cook:

- Cook the pancakes until bubbles form on the surface, then flip and cook the other side until golden brown.

Repeat:

- Repeat the process until all the batter is used, adding more butter or oil to the pan as needed.

Serve Warm:

- Serve the cottage cheese pancakes warm. They can be enjoyed on their own or with toppings of your choice, such as fresh berries, sugar-free syrup, or a dollop of whipped cream.

Optional Garnishes:

- Get creative with garnishes! Consider adding a sprinkle of cinnamon, a drizzle of honey, or a handful of chopped nuts for extra flavor and texture.

Enjoy:

- Enjoy these delightful cottage cheese pancakes as a nutritious and satisfying breakfast or brunch option. They are not only delicious but also provide a good balance of protein and low-carb goodness.

Baked Apple Oatmeal

Ingredients:

- 2 cups old-fashioned oats
- 1/2 cup chopped nuts (walnuts or pecans work well)
- 1 teaspoon baking powder
- 1 1/2 teaspoons ground cinnamon
- 1/4 teaspoon salt
- 2 cups milk (dairy or plant-based)

- 1/4 cup maple syrup or honey
- 2 large eggs
- 2 teaspoons vanilla extract
- 2 medium-sized apples, peeled, cored, and diced
- Butter or oil for greasing the baking dish

Servings: 6-8

Instructions:

- Preheat your oven to 350°F (175°C). Grease a baking dish with butter or oil.
- In a large mixing bowl, combine the old-fashioned oats, chopped nuts, baking powder, ground cinnamon, and salt. Mix well until the dry ingredients are evenly distributed.
- In another bowl, whisk together the milk, maple syrup or honey, eggs, and vanilla extract until well combined.
- Pour the wet ingredients into the bowl of dry ingredients. Stir until everything is well incorporated.
- Gently fold in the diced apples, ensuring they are evenly distributed throughout the mixture.
- Pour the oatmeal mixture into the greased baking dish, spreading it out evenly.
- Bake in the preheated oven for 35-40 minutes or until the top is golden brown, and the oatmeal is set.
- Allow the baked apple oatmeal to cool for a few minutes before slicing and serving. You can serve it warm with a dollop of yogurt, a drizzle of maple syrup, or additional fresh fruit if desired.
- Store any leftovers in an airtight container in the refrigerator. This baked apple oatmeal reheats well, making it a convenient option for busy mornings.

Breakfast Burrito Bowl

Ingredients:

- 2 cups cauliflower rice
- 1 tablespoon olive oil
- 1/2 cup diced bell peppers (assorted colors)
- 1/2 cup diced red onion
- 1 cup cooked and seasoned ground turkey or chicken
- 1/2 avocado, sliced
- 1/4 cup salsa
- 2 tablespoons chopped fresh cilantro
- Salt and pepper to taste

Servings: 2

Instructions:

- In a food processor, pulse cauliflower florets until they resemble rice grains.
- In a pan, heat olive oil over medium heat. Add cauliflower rice and sauté for 5-7 minutes, or until tender. Season with salt and pepper, to taste.
- In the same pan, add diced bell peppers and red onion. Sauté until vegetables are tender but still have a slight crunch.
- In a separate pan, cook ground turkey or chicken over medium heat until fully cooked. Season with your favorite spices, such as cumin, chili powder, garlic powder, and salt.
- Divide the cauliflower rice among two bowls.
- Top with the cooked ground turkey or chicken, sautéed vegetables, sliced avocado, salsa, and chopped cilantro.
- Mix the ingredients in the bowl to combine flavors.
- Garnish with extra cilantro and a wedge of lime, if desired.
- Serve immediately and savor the delicious flavors of this satisfying breakfast burrito bowl.

Almond Flour Banana Muffins

Ingredients:

- 2 ripe bananas, mashed
- 3 large eggs
- 1/4 cup melted coconut oil or butter
- 1 teaspoon vanilla extract
- 2 cups almond flour
- 1/2 teaspoon baking soda
- 1/4 teaspoon salt
- Optional: Chopped nuts or dark chocolate chips for added texture

Servings: Makes approximately 12 muffins.

Instructions:

- Preheat your oven to 350°F (175°C). Line a muffin tin with paper liners or grease the cups.
- In a large mixing bowl, combine the mashed bananas, eggs, melted coconut oil or butter, and vanilla extract. Mix until well combined.
- In a separate bowl, whisk together the almond flour, baking soda, and salt.
- Gradually add the dry ingredients to the wet ingredients, stirring until a batter forms. Mix until there are no visible lumps.
- If desired, fold in chopped nuts or dark chocolate chips for added flavor and texture.
- Spoon the batter into the prepared muffin cups, filling each about 2/3 full.
- Bake in the preheated oven for 20-25 minutes or until a toothpick inserted into the center of a muffin comes out clean.

- Allow the muffins to cool in the tin for a few minutes before transferring them to a wire rack to cool completely.
- Once cooled, these almond flour banana muffins are ready to be enjoyed. Serve with your favorite beverage and savor the delightful combination of almond and banana flavors.

Salmon and Dill Frittata

Ingredients:
- 6 large eggs
- 1/2 cup smoked salmon, chopped
- 1/4 cup fresh dill, chopped
- 1/2 cup cream or milk
- 1/2 cup cream cheese, softened
- Salt and pepper to taste
- 2 tablespoons butter for greasing

Servings: 4

Instructions:
- Preheat your oven broiler.
- In a bowl, whisk together the eggs, cream or milk, and softened cream cheese until well combined. Season with salt and pepper to taste.
- In an oven-safe skillet, melt the butter over medium heat.
- Add the chopped smoked salmon and fresh dill to the skillet, sautéing for 2-3 minutes until the salmon is slightly cooked.
- Pour the whisked egg mixture over the sautéed salmon and dill in the skillet. Allow it to set for a minute without stirring.
- Cook on the stovetop for 3-4 minutes, gently lifting the edges to let any uncooked egg flow underneath.
- Once the edges are set, transfer the skillet to the preheated broiler. Broil for 3-5 minutes or until the top is golden and the frittata is puffed.
- Carefully remove the skillet from the oven using oven mitts.
- Allow the frittata to cool for a minute, then slice it into wedges.
- Serve warm and garnish with additional fresh dill if desired.
- Enjoy your Salmon and Dill Frittata as a delightful breakfast or brunch option. Pair it with a side salad for a complete and satisfying meal.

Coconut Flour Waffles

Ingredients:
- 1 cup coconut flour
- 1 teaspoon baking powder
- 1/4 teaspoon salt

- 4 large eggs
- 1 cup coconut milk
- 2 tablespoons coconut oil, melted
- 1 teaspoon vanilla extract

Servings: Makes approximately 4-6 waffles, depending on the size of your waffle maker.

Instructions:
- Turn on your waffle maker and let it preheat according to the manufacturer's instructions.
- In a large mixing bowl, whisk together the coconut flour, baking powder, and salt until well combined.
- In a separate bowl, beat the eggs. Add the coconut milk, melted coconut oil, and vanilla extract. Mix well.
- Pour the wet ingredients into the bowl with the dry ingredients. Stir until you have a smooth batter. The coconut flour may absorb moisture, so let the batter sit for a couple of minutes to thicken.
- Lightly grease the waffle maker with coconut oil or non-stick cooking spray.
- Pour an appropriate amount of batter onto the preheated waffle maker. Close the lid and cook according to the manufacturer's instructions, usually for about 4-5 minutes, until the waffles are golden brown and crisp.
- Carefully remove the waffles from the maker and place them on a serving plate.
- Serve the coconut flour waffles warm with your favorite toppings such as fresh berries, coconut flakes, or a drizzle of sugar-free syrup.
- Get creative with your toppings! Consider adding whipped coconut cream, chopped nuts, or a sprinkle of cinnamon for extra flavor.
- Relish in the delightful and slightly sweet flavor of these coconut flour waffles, perfect for a wholesome and satisfying breakfast.

Turkey and Vegetable Breakfast Skillet

Ingredients:
- 1 pound ground turkey
- 1 tablespoon olive oil
- 1 small onion, diced
- 1 bell pepper, diced (any color)
- 1 zucchini, diced
- 2 cloves garlic, minced
- Salt and pepper to taste
- 1 teaspoon dried oregano
- 1 teaspoon paprika
- 4 large eggs
- Fresh parsley for garnish (optional)

Servings: 4 servings

Instructions:
- In a large skillet, heat olive oil over medium heat. Add the ground turkey and cook until browned, breaking it apart with a spoon as it cooks.
- Add diced onion, bell pepper, and zucchini to the skillet. Sauté until the vegetables are softened, and the onion is translucent.
- Stir in minced garlic, dried oregano, paprika, salt, and pepper. Combine well, allowing the flavors to meld for a couple of minutes.
- Make four wells in the vegetable and turkey mixture using the back of a spoon. Crack an egg into each well, ensuring they are evenly spaced.
- Cover the skillet and cook until the egg whites are set but the yolks are still runny, about 5-7 minutes. Adjust the cooking time if you prefer firmer yolks.
- Sprinkle fresh parsley over the top for added freshness and color. Serve the breakfast skillet hot, directly from the pan.
- Optional: Toasted Bread or Tortillas, Accompany the skillet with your choice of toasted whole-grain bread or tortillas for a complete and satisfying breakfast.
- Dive into a flavorful and protein-packed breakfast that combines the goodness of turkey and a variety of colorful vegetables. Adjust the seasonings to your liking and savor this nutritious start to your day!

Mushroom and Spinach Egg Cups

Ingredients:
- 1 cup mushrooms, finely chopped
- 1 cup fresh spinach, chopped
- 6 large eggs
- 1/4 cup heavy cream
- 1/2 cup shredded mozzarella cheese
- 2 tablespoons unsalted butter
- Salt and pepper to taste
- Fresh chives, chopped (for garnish, optional)

Servings: 6 Egg Cups

Instructions:
- Preheat your oven to 375°F (190°C). Grease a muffin tin with butter or cooking spray to prevent sticking.
- In a skillet over medium heat, melt the butter. Add finely chopped mushrooms and cook until they release their moisture, about 5 minutes.
- Add chopped spinach to the skillet and sauté until wilted. Season with salt and pepper to taste. Set aside to cool.

- In a mixing bowl, whisk together the eggs and heavy cream until well combined. Season with a pinch of salt and pepper.
- Distribute the mushroom and spinach mixture evenly among the greased muffin tin cups.
- Pour the egg mixture over the vegetables in each cup, filling about 3/4 of the way. Sprinkle shredded mozzarella on top.
- Place the muffin tin in the preheated oven and bake for 15-18 minutes or until the eggs are set and slightly golden on top.
- Once cooked, remove the egg cups from the oven and let them cool for a few minutes.
- If desired, garnish with fresh chopped chives for added flavor and presentation.
- Carefully remove the egg cups from the muffin tin using a spatula. Serve them warm and enjoy a nutritious and delicious breakfast or brunch option!

Protein-Packed Smoothie Bowl

Ingredients:
- 1 cup unsweetened almond milk
- 1 scoop vanilla protein powder
- 1/2 frozen banana
- 1/2 cup frozen mixed berries
- 1 tablespoon almond butter
- 1 tablespoon chia seeds
- Toppings: sliced strawberries, blueberries, granola, and a drizzle of honey (optional)

Servings: 1

Instructions:
- Place the unsweetened almond milk, vanilla protein powder, frozen banana, frozen mixed berries, almond butter, and chia seeds into a blender.
- Blend the ingredients on high speed until you achieve a smooth and creamy consistency. Make sure all the frozen fruits are well incorporated.
- Adjust the thickness by adding more almond milk if necessary. The goal is to achieve a thick, spoonable consistency.
- Pour the smoothie mixture into a bowl, ensuring an even distribution.
- Sprinkle sliced strawberries, blueberries, and granola on top for added texture and flavor. Drizzle with honey if desired.
- Get creative with additional toppings such as shredded coconut, chopped nuts, or a dollop of Greek yogurt.
- Enjoy your protein-packed smoothie bowl immediately to savor the freshness and optimal texture.

Peanut Butter and Banana Toast

Ingredients:
- 2 slices of whole-grain bread
- 2 tablespoons of natural peanut butter
- 1 ripe banana, sliced
- Honey (optional, for drizzling)

Servings: 2 servings

Instructions:
- Place the slices of whole-grain bread in a toaster or toaster oven.
- Toast the bread to your desired level of crispiness.
- Once the bread is toasted, spread a generous layer of natural peanut butter on each slice. Ensure an even coating for a satisfying taste in every bite.
- Arrange the banana slices on top of the peanut butter-covered bread. You can place them in a neat pattern or scatter them for an artistic touch.
- If you desire a touch of sweetness, drizzle honey over the banana slices. This step is optional and can be adjusted based on your preference for sweetness.
- Place the prepared slices on a plate and savor the delightful combination of creamy peanut butter, sweet banana, and, if added, the hint of honey.
- This Peanut Butter and Banana Toast makes for a satisfying breakfast, quick snack, or energy-boosting pre-workout treat.
- Explore variations by adding a sprinkle of chia seeds, a dash of cinnamon, or a handful of chopped nuts for extra texture and flavor.

Cauliflower Hash Browns

Ingredients:
- 1 medium-sized cauliflower head, grated
- 1/2 cup grated Parmesan cheese
- 1/4 cup almond flour
- 2 large eggs
- 1/2 teaspoon garlic powder
- 1/2 teaspoon onion powder
- Salt and pepper to taste
- Cooking oil for frying

Servings: 4 servings

Instructions:
- Wash and dry the cauliflower head thoroughly.
- Grate the cauliflower using a box grater or a food processor until it resembles rice.
- Place the grated cauliflower in a clean kitchen towel or cheesecloth.

- Squeeze out excess moisture from the cauliflower. This step is crucial to achieving crispy hash browns.
- In a large mixing bowl, combine the grated cauliflower, Parmesan cheese, almond flour, eggs, garlic powder, onion powder, salt, and pepper.
- Mix well until all the ingredients are evenly incorporated.
- Take a portion of the mixture and shape it into a round patty, pressing firmly to hold its shape.
- Repeat the process until all the mixture is used, creating uniform-sized hash brown patties.
- Heat a skillet or frying pan over medium heat and add a thin layer of cooking oil.
- Carefully place the cauliflower hash browns in the pan, making sure not to overcrowd.
- Cook for 3-4 minutes on each side, or until golden brown and crispy.
- Once cooked, transfer the hash browns to a plate lined with paper towels to absorb any excess oil.
- Serve the cauliflower hash browns immediately while they are hot and crispy.
- Optionally, garnish with fresh herbs or serve with your favorite dipping sauce.
- Relish the delicious, low-carb alternative to traditional hash browns, guilt-free and full of flavor!

Mango and Lime Overnight Oats

Ingredients:
- 1 cup rolled oats
- 1 cup unsweetened almond milk (or any milk of your choice)
- 1 ripe mango, diced
- 1 tablespoon chia seeds
- Zest of one lime
- 1-2 tablespoons lime juice
- 1-2 tablespoons honey or maple syrup (optional, depending on sweetness preference)

Servings: Makes 2 servings

Instructions:
- In a bowl, combine the rolled oats and almond milk. Stir well to ensure the oats are fully coated. This forms the base of your overnight oats.
- Sprinkle chia seeds into the oat mixture. Chia seeds will absorb liquid and add a pleasant, pudding-like texture to your oats.
- If desired, add honey or maple syrup to sweeten the oats. Adjust the sweetness according to your preference.
- Gently fold in the diced mango, distributing it evenly throughout the oat mixture. The ripe mango adds natural sweetness and a tropical flavor.

- Grate the zest of one lime directly into the oats for a burst of citrus flavor. Squeeze lime juice into the mixture, adjusting the quantity based on your taste preferences.
- Thoroughly mix all the ingredients to ensure an even distribution of flavors. Make sure the oats and chia seeds are well combined.
- Divide the mixture into two airtight jars or containers. Seal tightly and refrigerate overnight or for at least 4-6 hours. This allows the oats and chia seeds to absorb the liquid and create a creamy, ready-to-eat texture.
- Once chilled, give the oats a final stir and taste. Adjust sweetness or add more lime juice if desired. Serve the Mango and Lime Overnight Oats chilled and enjoy a refreshing, nutritious breakfast or snack.

Grilled Chicken and Vegetable Skewers

Ingredients:
- 1 pound boneless, skinless chicken breasts, cut into bite-sized cubes
- 1 zucchini, sliced into rounds
- 1 red bell pepper, cut into chunks
- 1 yellow bell pepper, cut into chunks
- 1 red onion, peeled and cut into wedges
- Cherry tomatoes
- Olive oil
- Garlic powder
- Dried oregano
- Salt and pepper, to taste
- Wooden skewers, soaked in water for at least 30 minutes

Servings: 4

Instructions:
- In a bowl, combine olive oil, garlic powder, dried oregano, salt, and pepper. Mix well to create the marinade.
- Place the chicken cubes in a separate bowl and coat them evenly with half of the marinade. Cover and let it marinate in the refrigerator for at least 30 minutes.
- In another bowl, toss the zucchini, red bell pepper, yellow bell pepper, red onion, and cherry tomatoes with the remaining marinade.
- Thread the marinated chicken and mixed vegetables alternately onto the soaked wooden skewers.
- Preheat the grill to medium-high heat.
- Place the skewers on the preheated grill and cook for about 10-15 minutes, turning occasionally, until the chicken is cooked through and the vegetables are tender and slightly charred.
- Once cooked, transfer the skewers to a serving platter. Optionally, garnish with fresh herbs like parsley or cilantro.
- Serve the grilled chicken and vegetable skewers hot, either as a standalone dish or over a bed of cooked rice or quinoa.

Mediterranean Quinoa Salad

Ingredients:
- 1 cup quinoa, rinsed and cooked
- 1 cup cherry tomatoes, halved

- 1 cucumber, diced
- 1/2 cup Kalamata olives, sliced
- 1/2 cup feta cheese, crumbled
- 1/4 cup red onion, finely chopped
- 1/4 cup fresh parsley, chopped

For the Dressing:
- 1/4 cup extra-virgin olive oil
- 2 tablespoons red wine vinegar
- 1 clove garlic, minced
- 1 teaspoon dried oregano
- Salt and black pepper to taste

Servings:
4-6 servings

Instructions:
Cook Quinoa:
- Rinse 1 cup of quinoa under cold water. In a saucepan, combine quinoa with 2 cups of water. Bring to a boil, then reduce heat, cover, and simmer for 15 minutes or until quinoa is cooked and water is absorbed. Let it cool.

Prepare Vegetables:
- In a large mixing bowl, combine the cooled quinoa, cherry tomatoes, diced cucumber, sliced Kalamata olives, crumbled feta cheese, finely chopped red onion, and fresh parsley.

Make the Dressing:
- In a small bowl, whisk together extra-virgin olive oil, red wine vinegar, minced garlic, dried oregano, salt, and black pepper. Adjust the seasoning to taste.

Combine and Toss:
- Pour the dressing over the quinoa and vegetable mixture. Gently toss everything together until well combined and evenly coated with the dressing.

Chill and Serve:
- Refrigerate the Mediterranean Quinoa Salad for at least 30 minutes before serving. This allows the flavors to meld. Serve chilled and enjoy as a refreshing and nutritious meal on its own or as a side dish.

Optional Garnish:
- Optionally, garnish with additional fresh parsley and a sprinkle of feta cheese before serving for an extra burst of flavor.

Salmon and Avocado Wrap

Ingredients:
- 2 salmon fillets
- 1 tablespoon olive oil
- Salt and pepper to taste
- 2 large whole-grain or low-carb wraps
- 1 ripe avocado, sliced
- 1 cup cherry tomatoes, halved
- 1/2 red onion, thinly sliced
- 1/4 cup Greek yogurt or sour cream
- Fresh cilantro or parsley for garnish

Servings: 2 wraps

Instructions:
- Preheat the oven to 400°F (200°C).
- Place the salmon fillets on a baking sheet.
- Drizzle with olive oil and season with salt and pepper.
- Bake for 12-15 minutes or until the salmon is cooked through and flakes easily with a fork.
- Lay out the whole-grain or low-carb wraps on a clean surface.
- Spread a layer of Greek yogurt or sour cream over each wrap.
- Place a salmon fillet in the center of each wrap.
- Add sliced avocado on top of the salmon.
- Sprinkle halved cherry tomatoes and thinly sliced red onion over the salmon and avocado.
- Garnish with fresh cilantro or parsley for added flavor.
- Carefully fold the sides of the wrap and then roll it up tightly, creating a secure wrap.
- Slice each wrap in half diagonally.
- Serve immediately and enjoy your delicious and nutritious Salmon and Avocado Wrap.

Cauliflower Fried Rice

Ingredients:

1 medium-sized cauliflower, riced
2 tablespoons vegetable oil
1 cup diced carrots
1 cup frozen peas
2 cloves garlic, minced
1/2 cup diced onion
2 eggs, beaten

3 tablespoons soy sauce (or tamari for a gluten-free option)
1 teaspoon sesame oil
2 green onions, thinly sliced
Salt and pepper to taste
Servings: 4

Instructions:

Prepare the Cauliflower Rice:
- Cut the cauliflower into florets and place them in a food processor.
- Pulse until the cauliflower resembles rice-like grains. Set aside.

Cook the Vegetables:
- In a large skillet or wok, heat 1 tablespoon of vegetable oil over medium heat.
- Add diced carrots and cook for 3-4 minutes until they start to soften.
- Stir in the frozen peas and cook for an additional 2-3 minutes.
- Push the vegetables to one side of the skillet.

Sauté Aromatics:
- In the cleared side of the skillet, add the remaining tablespoon of oil.
- Sauté minced garlic and diced onion until fragrant and translucent.

Cook the Cauliflower Rice:
- Add the riced cauliflower to the skillet with the sautéed vegetables.
- Stir well to combine and cook for 5-7 minutes, allowing the cauliflower to cook through.

Create a Well for Eggs:
- Push the cauliflower mixture to the sides of the skillet, creating a well in the center.
- Pour the beaten eggs into the well and scramble until cooked through.

Combine and Season:
- Mix the scrambled eggs with the cauliflower mixture.
- Pour soy sauce (or tamari) and sesame oil over the entire mixture.
- Stir well to ensure even distribution of flavors.
- Season with salt and pepper, to taste.

Finish and Garnish:
- Stir in sliced green onions.
- Continue cooking for an additional 2-3 minutes until everything is heated through.

Serve:
- Divide the cauliflower fried rice among serving plates.
- Garnish with additional green onions, if desired.
- Enjoy your delicious and low-carb cauliflower fried rice!

Turkey and Spinach Stuffed Peppers

Ingredients:

- 4 large bell peppers, halved and seeds removed
- 1 pound ground turkey
- 1 cup spinach, chopped
- 1 cup cauliflower rice
- 1 cup diced tomatoes
- 1/2 cup diced onions
- 2 cloves garlic, minced
- 1 teaspoon olive oil
- 1 teaspoon dried oregano
- 1 teaspoon ground cumin
- 1/2 teaspoon paprika
- Salt and pepper to taste
- 1 cup shredded mozzarella cheese (optional, for topping)

Servings: Makes 8 stuffed pepper halves

Instructions:

- Preheat your oven to 375°F (190°C).
- Cut the bell peppers in half lengthwise, and remove the seeds and membranes. Place the pepper halves in a baking dish.
- In a skillet over medium heat, add olive oil. Sauté the diced onions until translucent, then add minced garlic and cook for an additional 1-2 minutes.
- Add ground turkey to the skillet and cook until browned. Stir in chopped spinach, cauliflower rice, diced tomatoes, oregano, cumin, paprika, salt, and pepper. Cook for an additional 5-7 minutes until the spinach wilts and the mixture is well combined.
- Spoon the turkey and spinach mixture evenly into each bell pepper half, pressing down gently to pack the filling.
- Cover the baking dish with foil and bake in the preheated oven for 25-30 minutes, or until the peppers are tender.
- If desired, remove the foil, sprinkle shredded mozzarella cheese on top of each stuffed pepper, and return to the oven. Bake for an additional 5-7 minutes or until the cheese is melted and bubbly.
- Carefully remove the stuffed peppers from the oven and let them cool slightly before serving. Garnish with fresh herbs if desired.
- Serve these Turkey and Spinach Stuffed Peppers hot, and enjoy a delicious, low-carb, and nutrient-packed meal!

Veggie and Hummus Wrap

Ingredients:

- Whole-grain or gluten-free tortillas
- Hummus (store-bought or homemade)
- Fresh spinach leaves
- Thinly sliced cucumber
- Sliced tomatoes
- Sliced red bell pepper
- Sliced red onion
- Avocado, sliced
- Feta cheese, crumbled (optional)
- Olive oil, for drizzling (optional)
- Salt and pepper, to taste

Servings: 2 wraps

Instructions:

Prepare the Tortillas:

- If using store-bought tortillas, warm them according to the package instructions.
- If making your own wraps, cook them on a dry skillet over medium heat for about 20-30 seconds on each side until they are pliable.

Spread Hummus:

- Lay out each tortilla and spread a generous layer of hummus over the surface, leaving about a 1-inch border around the edges.

Layer the Vegetables:

- Arrange a handful of fresh spinach leaves over the hummus layer.
- Add a layer of thinly sliced cucumber, followed by sliced tomatoes, red bell pepper, red onion, and avocado slices.

Add Optional Ingredients:

- If desired, sprinkle crumbled feta cheese over the veggies.
- Drizzle with olive oil for added flavor.
- Season with salt and pepper to taste.

Wrap it Up:

- Begin wrapping the tortilla tightly from one side, folding in the edges as you go.
- Continue rolling until the entire wrap is enclosed.

Slice and Serve:

- Use a sharp knife to slice the wrap in half diagonally.
- Serve immediately, securing each half with toothpicks if needed.

Enjoy:

- Savor the vibrant flavors and textures of your Veggie and Hummus Wrap. This versatile and nutritious meal is perfect for a quick lunch or a light dinn

Chickpea and Tomato Salad

Ingredients:

- 1 can (15 oz) chickpeas, drained and rinsed
- 1 cup cherry tomatoes, halved
- 1/2 cucumber, diced
- 1/4 red onion, finely chopped
- 1/4 cup fresh parsley, chopped
- 2 tablespoons extra-virgin olive oil
- 1 tablespoon red wine vinegar
- Salt and pepper to taste

Servings: 4

Instructions:

- Drain and rinse the canned chickpeas thoroughly. Set aside.
- In a large mixing bowl, combine the chickpeas, cherry tomatoes, diced cucumber, chopped red onion, and fresh parsley.
- In a small bowl, whisk together the extra-virgin olive oil and red wine vinegar. Season with salt and pepper to taste.
- Pour the dressing over the chickpea and vegetable mixture. Gently toss the salad to ensure an even coating of the dressing.
- Chill (Optional):For enhanced flavor, refrigerate the salad for at least 30 minutes before serving. This allows the ingredients to marinate and the flavors to meld.
- Once chilled, or if you prefer it at room temperature, serve the Chickpea and Tomato Salad in individual bowls or as a side dish.
- Optional Additions:Customize the salad by adding crumbled feta cheese, olives, or a sprinkle of your favorite herbs for an extra burst of flavor.
- Garnish with additional parsley if desired, and enjoy this refreshing and nutritious Chickpea and Tomato Salad!

Eggplant and Zucchini Lasagna

Ingredients:

- 1 large eggplant, thinly sliced
- 2 medium-sized zucchinis, thinly sliced
- 1 pound ground beef or ground turkey
- 1 onion, finely chopped
- 3 cloves garlic, minced
- 1 can (14 ounces) crushed tomatoes
- 1 can (6 ounces) tomato paste
- 1 teaspoon dried oregano
- 1 teaspoon dried basil

- Salt and pepper to taste
- 2 cups ricotta cheese
- 1 large egg
- 2 cups shredded mozzarella cheese
- 1/2 cup grated Parmesan cheese
- Fresh basil leaves for garnish (optional)

Servings: 6-8

Instructions:
- Preheat your oven to 375°F (190°C).
- Place the sliced eggplant and zucchini on a baking sheet. Sprinkle them with salt and let them sit for about 15 minutes to draw out excess moisture. Pat them dry with a paper towel.
- In a large skillet over medium heat, brown the ground beef or turkey. Add chopped onions and minced garlic. Cook until the onions are translucent.
- Stir in the crushed tomatoes, tomato paste, dried oregano, dried basil, salt, and pepper. Simmer for about 10-15 minutes, allowing the flavors to meld.
- In a bowl, mix the ricotta cheese with one beaten egg until well combined.
- In a greased baking dish, layer the eggplant and zucchini slices. Spread half of the meat sauce over the vegetables. Dollop half of the ricotta mixture over the sauce. Sprinkle with mozzarella and Parmesan cheese. Repeat the layers.
- Cover the baking dish with foil and bake in the preheated oven for 30 minutes. Then, remove the foil and bake for an additional 15-20 minutes, or until the cheese is golden and bubbly.
- Allow the lasagna to rest for 10 minutes before slicing. Garnish with fresh basil leaves if desired.
- Serve the Eggplant and Zucchini Lasagna warm, and enjoy a delicious, low-carb alternative to traditional lasagna.

Tofu Stir-Fry with Broccoli and Bell Peppers

Ingredients:
- 1 block of firm tofu, pressed and cubed
- 2 cups broccoli florets
- 1 red bell pepper, thinly sliced
- 1 yellow bell pepper, thinly sliced
- 3 tablespoons soy sauce (or tamari for a gluten-free option)
- 2 tablespoons sesame oil
- 1 tablespoon rice vinegar
- 1 tablespoon maple syrup or sweetener of choice
- 2 cloves garlic, minced

- 1 teaspoon ginger, grated
- 2 tablespoons vegetable oil (for stir-frying)
- Sesame seeds and green onions for garnish (optional)
- Cooked rice or noodles for serving

Servings: 4

Instructions:
- Place the block of tofu on a plate lined with paper towels. Cover with more paper towels and place a heavy object on top (such as a can or a skillet). Press for at least 15-20 minutes to remove excess moisture.
- Once pressed, cut the tofu into bite-sized cubes.
- Cut broccoli into small florets.
- Thinly slice the red and yellow bell peppers.
- In a small bowl, whisk together soy sauce, sesame oil, rice vinegar, maple syrup, minced garlic, and grated ginger. Set aside.
- Heat 1 tablespoon of vegetable oil in a large skillet or wok over medium-high heat.
- Add tofu cubes and cook until golden brown on all sides. Remove tofu from the pan and set aside.
- In the same pan, add another tablespoon of vegetable oil.
- Stir-fry broccoli and bell peppers until they are slightly tender but still vibrant, about 4-5 minutes.
- Return the cooked tofu to the pan with the vegetables.
- Pour the stir-fry sauce over the tofu and vegetables. Toss everything together until well-coated and heated through.
- Serve the tofu stir-fry over cooked rice or noodles.
- Garnish with sesame seeds and sliced green onions if desired.
- Dive into a delicious and nutritious Tofu Stir-Fry with Broccoli and Bell Peppers, balancing flavors and textures in every bite.

Spinach and Feta Stuffed Chicken Breast

Ingredients:
- 4 boneless, skinless chicken breasts
- 2 cups fresh spinach, chopped
- 1 cup crumbled feta cheese
- 2 cloves garlic, minced
- 1 tablespoon olive oil
- 1 teaspoon dried oregano
- Salt and pepper to taste
- Toothpicks or kitchen twine (for securing the chicken)

Servings: 4

Instructions:

- Preheat your oven to 375°F (190°C).
- In a skillet over medium heat, sauté the chopped spinach and minced garlic in olive oil until the spinach wilts. Remove from heat and let it cool.
- In a bowl, combine the sautéed spinach mixture with crumbled feta cheese. Add dried oregano, salt, and pepper to taste. Mix well.
- Lay the chicken breasts flat on a clean surface. Using a sharp knife, make a horizontal cut along the side of each chicken breast to create a pocket without cutting all the way through.
- Stuff each chicken breast pocket with the spinach and feta mixture. Secure the openings with toothpicks or tie with kitchen twine to keep the filling intact.
- Season the stuffed chicken breasts with salt, pepper, and a sprinkle of additional dried oregano if desired.
- In an oven-safe skillet, heat olive oil over medium-high heat. Sear the stuffed chicken breasts on each side until golden brown, about 2-3 minutes per side.
- Transfer the skillet to the preheated oven and bake for 20-25 minutes or until the chicken reaches an internal temperature of 165°F (74°C).
- Allow the stuffed chicken breasts to rest for a few minutes before removing toothpicks or twine. Slice and serve with your favorite side dishes.
- Enjoy your delicious Spinach and Feta Stuffed Chicken Breast!

Black Bean and Corn Salad

Ingredients:

- 1 can (15 ounces) black beans, drained and rinsed
- 1 cup frozen corn kernels, thawed
- 1 cup cherry tomatoes, halved
- 1/2 red onion, finely diced
- 1/4 cup fresh cilantro, chopped
- 1 avocado, diced
- 2 tablespoons olive oil
- 1 lime, juiced
- Salt and pepper to taste

Servings:

4 servings

Instructions:

Prepare the Ingredients:

- Drain and rinse the black beans thoroughly.
- Thaw the frozen corn kernels and ensure they are at room temperature.

- Halve the cherry tomatoes.
- Finely dice the red onion.
- Chop the fresh cilantro.
- Dice the avocado.

Combine Ingredients in a Bowl:
- In a large mixing bowl, combine the black beans, corn kernels, cherry tomatoes, red onion, cilantro, and diced avocado.

Make the Dressing:
- In a small bowl, whisk together the olive oil and lime juice. Adjust the ratio to taste, adding more lime juice if desired.
- Season the dressing with salt and pepper to taste.

Dress the Salad:
- Pour the dressing over the black bean and corn mixture. Gently toss the salad to ensure even coating.

Chill and Marinate (Optional):
For enhanced flavor, cover the bowl and refrigerate the salad for at least 30 minutes to allow the flavors to meld. This step is optional but recommended for a more refreshing taste.

Serve:
- Once chilled (if preferred), serve the black bean and corn salad in individual bowls or as a side dish.

Optional Garnish:
- Garnish with additional cilantro leaves or avocado slices if desired.

Enjoy:
- This Black Bean and Corn Salad is now ready to be enjoyed as a light and flavorful dish. Serve it on its own or as a side dish with grilled chicken or fish.

Shrimp and Asparagus Quiche

Ingredients:
- 1 lb (450g) shrimp, peeled and deveined
- 1 bunch asparagus, trimmed and chopped
- 1 cup cherry tomatoes, halved
- 1 cup shredded Gruyère or Swiss cheese
- 1 tablespoon olive oil
- 1 teaspoon garlic powder
- 1 teaspoon dried thyme
- Salt and pepper to taste
- 6 large eggs
- 1 cup heavy cream

Servings: 6-8 servings

Instructions:

Preheat the Oven:

- Preheat your oven to 375°F (190°C). Grease a pie or quiche dish.

Prepare the Shrimp and Vegetables:

- In a skillet over medium heat, heat olive oil.
- Add shrimp and cook until pink and opaque, about 2-3 minutes per side. Remove shrimp from the skillet and set aside.
- In the same skillet, add chopped asparagus and sauté until tender-crisp, about 3-4 minutes.
- Season asparagus with garlic powder, dried thyme, salt, and pepper. Remove from heat.

Assemble the Quiche:

- In the prepared pie or quiche dish, arrange the cooked shrimp, asparagus, and halved cherry tomatoes.
- Sprinkle shredded Gruyère or Swiss cheese evenly over the ingredients.

Prepare the Egg Mixture:

- In a bowl, whisk together eggs and heavy cream until well combined. Season with salt and pepper to taste.

Pour the Egg Mixture:

- Pour the egg mixture over the shrimp, asparagus, tomatoes, and cheese in the dish. Ensure an even distribution.

Bake the Quiche:

- Place the quiche dish in the preheated oven and bake for 30-35 minutes or until the eggs are set and the top is golden brown.

Serve:

- Allow the quiche to cool for a few minutes before slicing.
- Serve warm and enjoy this delightful Shrimp and Asparagus Quiche for brunch or a light dinner.

Optional Garnish:

- Garnish with fresh herbs, such as chopped parsley or chives, for added flavor and visual appeal.

Turkey and Vegetable Skillet

Ingredients:

- 1 lb ground turkey
- 1 tablespoon olive oil
- 1 onion, finely chopped
- 2 cloves garlic, minced
- 1 bell pepper, diced (you can use a mix of colors for visual appeal)
- 1 zucchini, diced

- 1 cup cherry tomatoes, halved
- 1 teaspoon dried oregano
- 1 teaspoon dried basil
- Salt and pepper to taste
- 1/2 cup shredded mozzarella cheese (optional, for topping)
- Fresh parsley, chopped (for garnish)

Instructions:
- Heat olive oil in a large skillet over medium heat.
- Add ground turkey, breaking it up with a spatula, and cook until browned.
- Add chopped onions and minced garlic to the skillet. Sauté until the onions are translucent and the garlic is fragrant.
- Stir in diced bell pepper and zucchini. Cook for a few minutes until the vegetables start to soften.
- Sprinkle dried oregano, dried basil, salt, and pepper over the turkey and vegetables. Mix well to distribute the seasonings evenly.
- Gently fold in the halved cherry tomatoes. Cook for an additional 3-5 minutes until the tomatoes are heated through but still retain their shape.
- If desired, sprinkle shredded mozzarella cheese over the skillet. Cover with a lid and let it melt for a couple of minutes.
- Once the cheese is melted (if using), garnish with fresh chopped parsley.
- Serve the turkey and vegetable skillet hot, either on its own or over cooked quinoa, rice, or pasta.

Sweet Potato and Chickpea Buddha Bowl

Ingredients:
- For the Buddha Bowl:
- 1 large sweet potato, peeled and cubed
- 1 can (15 oz) chickpeas, drained and rinsed
- 1 tablespoon olive oil
- 1 teaspoon smoked paprika
- 1 teaspoon cumin
- Salt and pepper to taste

For the Bowl Assembly:
- Cooked quinoa or brown rice
- Mixed greens (e.g., spinach, kale, arugula)
- Cherry tomatoes, halved
- Cucumber, sliced
- Avocado, sliced
- Red onion, thinly sliced
- Hummus for topping
- Lemon wedges for garnish

Instructions:

- Preheat the oven to 400°F (200°C).
- In a bowl, toss the sweet potato cubes and chickpeas with olive oil, smoked paprika, cumin, salt, and pepper until evenly coated.
- Spread the sweet potatoes and chickpeas on a baking sheet in a single layer.
- Roast in the oven for about 25-30 minutes or until sweet potatoes are tender and chickpeas are crispy.
- While the sweet potatoes and chickpeas are roasting, cook quinoa or brown rice according to package instructions.
- In individual bowls, start with a base of cooked quinoa or brown rice.
- Arrange a portion of roasted sweet potatoes and chickpeas on top.
- Add a handful of mixed greens, cherry tomatoes, cucumber slices, avocado slices, and red onion.
- Drizzle each bowl with a spoonful of hummus.
- Garnish with lemon wedges for a fresh squeeze before serving.
- Mix the ingredients in the bowl before eating or enjoy each component separately.
- Adjust seasoning and add extra olive oil or lemon juice if desired.

Greek Chicken Souvlaki Salad

Ingredients:

For the Chicken Souvlaki:

- 1.5 lbs boneless, skinless chicken breasts, cut into cubes
- 3 tablespoons olive oil
- 3 tablespoons Greek yogurt
- 3 cloves garlic, minced
- 1 teaspoon dried oregano
- 1 teaspoon dried thyme
- 1 teaspoon paprika
- Juice of 1 lemon
- Salt and pepper to taste

For the Salad:

- Mixed salad greens (lettuce, spinach, arugula, etc.)
- Cherry tomatoes, halved
- Cucumber, sliced
- Red onion, thinly sliced
- Kalamata olives, pitted
- Feta cheese, crumbled

For the Dressing:
- 1/4 cup extra virgin olive oil
- 2 tablespoons red wine vinegar
- 1 teaspoon Dijon mustard
- 1 teaspoon dried oregano
- Salt and pepper to taste

Instructions:
- In a bowl, combine olive oil, Greek yogurt, minced garlic, dried oregano, dried thyme, paprika, lemon juice, salt, and pepper. Mix well to create the marinade.
- Add the chicken cubes to the marinade, ensuring they are well coated. Cover the bowl and let it marinate in the refrigerator for at least 30 minutes, or preferably a few hours to allow the flavors to meld.
- Preheat a grill or grill pan over medium-high heat. Thread the marinated chicken cubes onto skewers.
- Grill the chicken skewers for about 6-8 minutes, turning occasionally, until the chicken is cooked through and has a nice char.
- While the chicken is grilling, prepare the salad by combining mixed greens, cherry tomatoes, cucumber, red onion, Kalamata olives, and feta cheese in a large bowl.
- In a small bowl, whisk together the ingredients for the dressing: olive oil, red wine vinegar, Dijon mustard, dried oregano, salt, and pepper.
- Once the chicken is done, remove it from the skewers and place it on top of the salad.
- Drizzle the dressing over the salad and chicken, tossing gently to combine.
- Serve immediately, garnished with additional feta cheese and olives if desired.

Lentil and Vegetable Curry

Ingredients:
- 1 cup dry lentils (green or brown), rinsed and drained
- 2 tablespoons vegetable oil
- 1 large onion, finely chopped
- 3 cloves garlic, minced
- 1 tablespoon ginger, grated
- 1 tablespoon curry powder
- 1 teaspoon ground cumin
- 1 teaspoon ground coriander
- 1/2 teaspoon turmeric
- 1/2 teaspoon chili powder (adjust to taste)
- 1 can (14 oz) diced tomatoes
- 1 can (14 oz) coconut milk
- 2 cups mixed vegetables (e.g., carrots, bell peppers, cauliflower, peas), chopped

- Salt and pepper to taste
- Fresh cilantro, chopped (for garnish)

Instructions:
- In a large pot, combine the lentils with enough water to cover them by about 2 inches.
- Bring to a boil, then reduce the heat and simmer for 20-25 minutes or until lentils are tender but not mushy.
- Drain any excess water and set aside.
- In a large skillet or pot, heat the vegetable oil over medium heat.
- Add chopped onions and sauté until translucent.
- Add minced garlic and grated ginger, and sauté for an additional minute until fragrant.
- Stir in the curry powder, ground cumin, ground coriander, turmeric, and chili powder. Cook for 1-2 minutes to toast the spices.
- Pour in the diced tomatoes (with their juices) and coconut milk. Mix well and bring to a simmer.
- Add the mixed vegetables to the pot. Cook until the vegetables are tender but still have a bit of crunch.
- Add the cooked lentils to the pot. Stir well to combine all the ingredients.
- Season the curry with salt and pepper to taste. Adjust the spice level if needed.
- Garnish with freshly chopped cilantro.
- Serve the lentil and vegetable curry over rice or with naan bread.

Cabbage and Turkey Sauté

Ingredients:
- 1 pound ground turkey
- 1 small head of cabbage, shredded
- 1 onion, finely chopped
- 2 cloves garlic, minced
- 1 bell pepper, diced
- 2 tablespoons olive oil
- 1 teaspoon dried thyme
- 1 teaspoon paprika
- Salt and pepper to taste
- Optional: Red pepper flakes for some heat
- Fresh parsley for garnish

Instructions:
- Heat olive oil in a large skillet or pan over medium heat.
- Add chopped onion and minced garlic to the pan. Sauté until the onions are translucent and the garlic is fragrant.

- Add ground turkey to the pan. Break it apart with a spatula and cook until it's browned and cooked through.
- Stir in the diced bell pepper and shredded cabbage. Cook for a few minutes until the vegetables start to soften.
- Season the mixture with dried thyme, paprika, salt, and pepper. If you like a bit of heat, you can also add red pepper flakes at this point.
- Continue to cook, stirring occasionally, until the cabbage is tender but still has a bit of crunch. Be careful not to overcook it.
- Taste and adjust the seasoning if needed.
- Once everything is cooked through and well combined, remove the pan from heat.
- Serve the cabbage and turkey sauté hot, garnished with fresh parsley.

Cucumber and Avocado Gazpacho

Ingredients:
- 2 large cucumbers, peeled and chopped
- 2 ripe avocados, peeled and diced
- 1 green bell pepper, seeded and chopped
- 1 small red onion, finely chopped
- 2 cloves garlic, minced
- 4 cups tomato juice or V8 vegetable juice
- 1/4 cup red wine vinegar
- 1/4 cup olive oil
- Salt and pepper to taste
- Fresh cilantro or parsley for garnish
- Optional toppings: diced tomatoes, croutons, or a drizzle of olive oil

Instructions:
- In a blender or food processor, combine the chopped cucumbers, avocados, green bell pepper, red onion, and minced garlic. Blend until smooth.
- Add the tomato juice, red wine vinegar, and olive oil to the blender. Blend again until all the ingredients are well combined and the mixture is smooth.
- Season the gazpacho with salt and pepper to taste. You can start with a small amount and adjust according to your preferences.
- Chill the gazpacho in the refrigerator for at least 2 hours to allow the flavors to meld and the soup to become cold.
- Before serving, taste the gazpacho again and adjust the seasoning if needed.
- Ladle the chilled gazpacho into bowls. Garnish with fresh cilantro or parsley.
- If desired, add toppings such as diced tomatoes, croutons, or a drizzle of olive oil just before serving.
- Serve the cucumber and avocado gazpacho cold and enjoy the refreshing flavors.

Pesto Zoodle Bowl

Ingredients:
For the Pesto Sauce:
- 2 cups fresh basil leaves, packed
- 1/2 cup grated Parmesan cheese
- 1/2 cup pine nuts or walnuts
- 2 cloves garlic, peeled
- 1/2 cup extra-virgin olive oil
- Salt and pepper to taste

For the Zoodle Bowl:
- 4 medium-sized zucchini, spiralized into noodles
- Cherry tomatoes, halved
- Red bell pepper, thinly sliced
- Black olives, sliced
- Grilled chicken or shrimp (optional)
- Additional Parmesan cheese for garnish
- Fresh basil leaves for garnish

Instructions:
Make the Pesto Sauce:
- In a food processor, combine basil, Parmesan cheese, pine nuts (or walnuts), and garlic.
- Pulse until the ingredients are finely chopped.
- With the processor running, slowly pour in the olive oil until the pesto reaches your desired consistency.
- Season with salt and pepper to taste. Set aside.

Prepare the Zoodles:
- Use a spiralizer to turn the zucchini into noodles.
- Heat a large skillet over medium heat and add a little olive oil.
- Sauté the zucchini noodles for 2-3 minutes until they are just tender.

Assemble the Bowl:
- Toss the zucchini noodles with the pesto sauce until well coated.
- Divide the zoodles among serving bowls.
- Top with cherry tomatoes, red bell pepper slices, black olives, and grilled chicken or shrimp if using.
- Garnish with additional Parmesan cheese and fresh basil leaves.

Serve:
- Enjoy your Pesto Zoodle Bowl immediately, while the zucchini noodles are still warm and the flavors are fresh.

Stuffed Portobello Mushrooms

Ingredients:
- 4 large Portobello mushrooms
- 1 tablespoon olive oil
- 1 small onion, finely chopped
- 2 cloves garlic, minced
- 1 cup fresh spinach, chopped
- 1/2 cup breadcrumbs
- 1/4 cup grated Parmesan cheese
- 1/4 cup shredded mozzarella cheese
- Salt and pepper to taste
- Fresh herbs (such as parsley or thyme) for garnish (optional)

Instructions:
- Preheat your oven to 375°F (190°C).
- Clean the Portobello mushrooms by wiping them with a damp cloth. Remove the stems and scoop out the gills using a spoon.
- In a skillet, heat olive oil over medium heat. Add chopped onions and garlic and sauté until they become translucent.
- Add chopped spinach to the skillet and cook until wilted. Season with salt and pepper to taste.
- In a mixing bowl, combine the sautéed vegetables with breadcrumbs, Parmesan cheese, and mozzarella cheese. Mix well to form a stuffing mixture.
- Place the Portobello mushrooms on a baking sheet lined with parchment paper or lightly greased.
- Stuff each mushroom cap with the vegetable and cheese mixture, pressing it down gently.
- Bake in the preheated oven for about 20-25 minutes or until the mushrooms are tender and the stuffing is golden brown.
- If desired, garnish with fresh herbs before serving.

Simple Snacks

Cucumber Hummus Bites

Ingredients:

1 large cucumber
1 cup hummus (store-bought or homemade)
Cherry tomatoes, sliced (optional, for garnish)
Fresh parsley, chopped (optional, for garnish)
Olive oil (optional, for drizzling)
Salt and pepper to taste

Instructions
- Wash the cucumber thoroughly and peel it if desired. If the cucumber has large seeds, you can use a spoon to scoop them out.
- Slice the cucumber into rounds, each about 1/2 inch thick. If you prefer, you can also cut the cucumber into thicker slices or even lengthwise strips.
- Take each cucumber slice and place a dollop of hummus on top. You can use a small spoon, knife, or a piping bag to make it look more decorative.
- Optional: Garnish each cucumber and hummus bite with a slice of cherry tomato, a sprinkle of chopped fresh parsley, or a drizzle of olive oil.
- Season the bites with a pinch of salt and pepper to taste. You can also add other seasonings like paprika, cumin, or red pepper flakes for extra flavor.
- Arrange the Cucumber Hummus Bites on a serving platter. They can be served immediately, or you can refrigerate them for a short time before serving to keep them cool.
- These bites make a refreshing and satisfying snack or appetizer. Enjoy the combination of the cool cucumber and the creamy hummus!

Avocado and Tomato Salsa Cups

Ingredients:
- 2 ripe avocados, diced
- 1 cup cherry tomatoes, diced
- 1/4 cup red onion, finely chopped
- 1/4 cup fresh cilantro, chopped
- 1 jalapeño pepper, seeded and finely chopped (optional for heat)
- 1 clove garlic, minced
- Juice of 1 lime
- Salt and pepper to taste

- Tortilla chips or small taco shells for serving

Instructions:
- Dice the avocados and tomatoes into small, bite-sized pieces.
- Finely chop the red onion, cilantro, and jalapeño (if using).
- Mince the garlic.
- Juice the lime.
- In a mixing bowl, gently combine the diced avocados, cherry tomatoes, red onion, cilantro, jalapeño (if using), and minced garlic.
- Squeeze the juice of one lime over the avocado and tomato mixture. The lime juice not only adds a zesty flavor but also helps prevent the avocados from browning.
- Season the salsa with salt and pepper to taste. Mix well to ensure all ingredients are evenly coated.
- Cover the bowl with plastic wrap and refrigerate the salsa for at least 30 minutes to allow the flavors to meld.
- Spoon the chilled avocado and tomato salsa into small cups or bowls. You can also use halved bell peppers or endive leaves as cups.
- Serve the avocado and tomato salsa cups with tortilla chips or small taco shells. Alternatively, you can use them as a topping for grilled chicken or fish.
- Garnish with extra cilantro or lime wedges if desired.

Cheese and Veggie Kabobs

Ingredients:
- 1 block of your favorite cheese (cheddar, mozzarella, or feta work well), cut into cubes
- Cherry tomatoes
- Bell peppers (assorted colors), cut into chunks
- Zucchini, sliced
- Red onion, cut into wedges
- Mushrooms, cleaned and halved
- Olive oil
- Salt and pepper, to taste
- Fresh herbs (such as basil or parsley), chopped for garnish (optional)
- Wooden or metal skewers

Instructions:
- Cut the cheese into cubes.
- Clean and chop the vegetables into bite-sized pieces.
- If using wooden skewers, soak them in water for about 30 minutes to prevent burning.
- Thread the cheese cubes and assorted veggies onto the skewers, alternating for a colorful presentation.
- Brush the assembled kabobs with olive oil, and season with salt and pepper to taste.

- Grill the kabobs on a preheated grill or broil in the oven for about 8-10 minutes, turning occasionally until the vegetables are tender and the cheese has a nice melt.
- Remove from the heat and let them rest for a minute.
- Garnish with fresh herbs if desired.
- You can add a marinade before grilling for extra flavor. A simple marinade can be made with olive oil, minced garlic, lemon juice, and your favorite herbs.
- Serve the cheese and veggie kabobs as a delightful appetizer or as a side dish.

Spiced Roasted Chickpeas

Ingredients:
- 2 cans (15 ounces each) of chickpeas (garbanzo beans), drained and rinsed
- 2 tablespoons olive oil
- 1 teaspoon ground cumin
- 1 teaspoon ground coriander
- 1 teaspoon smoked paprika
- 1/2 teaspoon cayenne pepper (adjust to taste)
- 1/2 teaspoon garlic powder
- 1/2 teaspoon onion powder
- 1/2 teaspoon salt (adjust to taste)
- Freshly ground black pepper to taste

Instructions:
- Preheat your oven to 400°F (200°C).
- Rinse and drain the chickpeas thoroughly. Pat them dry with a paper towel to remove excess moisture. The drier they are, the crispier they will become.
- In a large bowl, combine the chickpeas with olive oil, cumin, coriander, smoked paprika, cayenne pepper, garlic powder, onion powder, salt, and black pepper. Toss until the chickpeas are evenly coated with the spices.
- Spread the seasoned chickpeas in a single layer on a baking sheet. Make sure they are not crowded enough to allow for even roasting.
- Roast in the preheated oven for about 25-30 minutes or until the chickpeas are golden brown and crispy. Shake the pan or stir the chickpeas halfway through the cooking time to ensure even roasting.
- Remove from the oven and let them cool for a few minutes. They will continue to crisp up as they cool.
- Taste and adjust the seasoning if necessary.
- Serve the spiced roasted chickpeas as a snack or use them as a crunchy topping for salads, soups, or yogurt.

Almond Butter-Stuffed Dates

Ingredients:
- Medjool dates (as many as you'd like to make)
- Almond butter (or any nut butter of your choice)
- Optional toppings: chopped nuts, shredded coconut, sea salt

Instructions:
- Use a knife to make a lengthwise slit in each date, removing the pit.
- Gently open the date to create a small pocket.
- Spoon a small amount of almond butter into each date. You can use smooth or crunchy almond butter based on your preference.
- If desired, roll the almond butter-stuffed dates in chopped nuts, shredded coconut, or sprinkle a bit of sea salt on top for added flavor and texture.
- Arrange the stuffed dates on a serving plate and enjoy! They make for a tasty and energy-boosting snack.
- You can get creative with variations by adding other ingredients like a sprinkle of cinnamon, a drizzle of honey, or even a touch of dark chocolate for an extra indulgence.
- Store any leftover stuffed dates in an airtight container in the refrigerator. They should stay fresh for several days.

Caprese Salad Skewers

Ingredients:
- Cherry tomatoes
- Fresh mozzarella balls (bocconcini)
- Fresh basil leaves
- Balsamic glaze
- Extra virgin olive oil
- Salt and pepper, to taste
- Wooden skewers

Instructions:
- Wash the cherry tomatoes and basil leaves.
- Drain the fresh mozzarella balls if they are stored in liquid.
- Take a wooden skewer and thread on a cherry tomato.
- Follow with a fresh basil leaf folded or rolled up, and then a mozzarella ball.
- Repeat the pattern until the skewer is filled, leaving some space at the ends for easy handling.
- Place the assembled Caprese Salad Skewers on a serving platter.
- Drizzle extra virgin olive oil over the skewers.
- Sprinkle salt and pepper to taste.

- Drizzle balsamic glaze over the skewers for a sweet and tangy flavor. You can create a balsamic reduction by simmering balsamic vinegar until it thickens, or you can use store-bought balsamic glaze.
- Arrange the skewers on a serving platter and serve immediately.

Tips:
- Use fresh and high-quality ingredients for the best flavor.
- If using wooden skewers, soak them in water for about 30 minutes before assembling to prevent them from burning.
- You can customize the size of the skewers based on your preference.
- Feel free to add a sprinkle of chopped fresh basil or a pinch of Italian herbs for extra flavor.

Guacamole Deviled Eggs

Ingredients:
- 6 hard-boiled eggs, peeled
- 2 ripe avocados
- 1 tablespoon lime juice
- 2 tablespoons finely chopped red onion
- 2 tablespoons diced tomatoes (seeds removed)
- 2 tablespoons chopped fresh cilantro
- 1 clove garlic, minced
- Salt and pepper to taste
- Paprika for garnish (optional)

Instructions:
- Place the eggs in a single layer in a saucepan.
- Cover the eggs with water, then bring to a boil.
- Once boiling, reduce heat to a simmer and let cook for 10-12 minutes.
- Transfer the eggs to an ice bath to cool, then peel and cut in half lengthwise.
- In a bowl, mash the avocados with a fork until smooth.
- Add lime juice, chopped red onion, diced tomatoes, cilantro, and minced garlic to the mashed avocados.
- Season with salt and pepper to taste.
- Mix everything together until well combined.
- Carefully remove the egg yolks from the halved eggs and place them in a separate bowl.
- Mash the egg yolks with a fork until they are smooth.
- Add the mashed egg yolks to the guacamole mixture.
- Mix until all ingredients are well incorporated.
- Spoon the guacamole and egg yolk mixture into the hollowed egg whites.

- You can use a spoon or a piping bag for a neater presentation.
- Optionally, sprinkle paprika on top of the filled eggs for a dash of color and flavor.
- Refrigerate the guacamole deviled eggs for at least 30 minutes before serving.
- Serve chilled and enjoy!

Cottage Cheese and Pineapple Cups

Ingredients:
- 1 cup cottage cheese
- 1 cup diced fresh pineapple
- 1 tablespoon honey (optional, for sweetness)
- 1/4 cup chopped fresh mint leaves (optional, for garnish)

Instructions:
- Cut a fresh pineapple in half lengthwise.
- Use a knife to carefully carve out the inside of each half, leaving a pineapple "bowl" or cup. Make sure to leave enough pineapple flesh on the sides to create a sturdy cup.
- Take the carved-out pineapple flesh and dice it into small, bite-sized pieces.
- In a mixing bowl, combine the cottage cheese with the diced pineapple.
- If you prefer a sweeter taste, drizzle honey over the cottage cheese and pineapple mixture. Adjust the amount according to your taste preference.
- Gently mix the cottage cheese, pineapple, and honey until well combined.
- Spoon the cottage cheese and pineapple mixture into the pineapple cups, filling them to the top.
- Sprinkle chopped fresh mint leaves over the top for a refreshing flavor and added visual appeal.
- Place the filled pineapple cups on a serving platter and serve immediately.

Turmeric Roasted Almonds

Ingredients:
- 2 cups whole almonds
- 1 tablespoon olive oil
- 1 teaspoon ground turmeric
- 1/2 teaspoon ground cumin
- 1/2 teaspoon paprika
- 1/2 teaspoon garlic powder
- 1/2 teaspoon onion powder
- 1/2 teaspoon salt (adjust to taste)
- 1/4 teaspoon black pepper (adjust to taste)

Instructions:

- Preheat your oven to 325°F (163°C).
- Place the almonds in a mixing bowl.
- Drizzle the olive oil over the almonds. Toss the almonds until they are evenly coated with the oil.
- In a small bowl, mix together the ground turmeric, ground cumin, paprika, garlic powder, onion powder, salt, and black pepper.
- Sprinkle the spice mixture over the almonds, ensuring they are well-coated. Toss the almonds until they are evenly covered with the spice mixture.
- Spread the seasoned almonds in a single layer on a baking sheet lined with parchment paper.
- Roast the almonds in the preheated oven for 15-20 minutes, stirring halfway through. Keep an eye on them to prevent burning.
- Once the almonds are golden brown and fragrant, remove them from the oven and let them cool completely on the baking sheet. They will continue to crisp up as they cool.
- Once completely cooled, transfer the turmeric roasted almonds to an airtight container. Store them at room temperature for up to two weeks.

Seaweed and Smoked Salmon Rolls

Ingredients:

- 4 sheets of nori seaweed
- 1 cup sushi rice, cooked and seasoned with rice vinegar, sugar, and salt
- 4 ounces smoked salmon, thinly sliced
- 1 cucumber, julienned
- 1 avocado, sliced
- Soy sauce, for dipping
- Pickled ginger and wasabi, for serving (optional)
- Sesame seeds, for garnish (optional)

Instructions:

- Cook sushi rice according to package instructions.
- While the rice is still warm, season it with a mixture of rice vinegar, sugar, and salt. Allow it to cool to room temperature.
- Slice the smoked salmon thinly.
- Julienne the cucumber.
- Slice the avocado.
- Place a sheet of nori seaweed on a bamboo sushi rolling mat.
- Wet your hands to prevent the rice from sticking and spread a thin layer of sushi rice over the nori, leaving about half an inch at the top.
- Arrange a few slices of smoked salmon, cucumber, and avocado horizontally on the rice.

- Carefully lift the edge of the bamboo mat closest to you, and begin rolling the seaweed and rice over the filling.
- Use the bamboo mat to shape the roll into a tight cylinder.
- Wet the exposed edge of the nori with a little water to seal the roll.
- Using a sharp knife, wet it with water to prevent sticking, and slice the roll into bite-sized pieces.
- Repeat the process with the remaining sheets of nori and ingredients.
- Arrange the sushi rolls on a plate.
- Sprinkle sesame seeds on top for garnish, if desired.
- Serve the rolls with soy sauce for dipping.
- Optionally, provide pickled ginger and wasabi on the side.

Berries and Ricotta Toast

Ingredients:
- 4 slices of your favorite bread (such as whole grain or sourdough)
- 1 cup fresh mixed berries (strawberries, blueberries, raspberries, etc.)
- 1 cup ricotta cheese
- 2 tablespoons honey (adjust to taste)
- Fresh mint leaves for garnish (optional)

Instructions:
- Toast the slices of bread to your desired level of crispiness. You can use a toaster, toaster oven, or a regular oven.
- Wash the berries thoroughly and pat them dry with a paper towel.
- If using strawberries, hull and slice them.
- Once the bread is toasted, spread a generous layer of ricotta cheese onto each slice.
- Place the fresh berries on top of the ricotta layer. You can arrange them neatly or scatter them, depending on your preference.
- Drizzle honey over the berries and ricotta. Adjust the amount according to your sweetness preference.
- If desired, garnish the toasts with fresh mint leaves for a burst of flavor and a touch of freshness.
- Place the prepared Berries and Ricotta Toasts on a serving plate and enjoy them immediately.

Zucchini Chips with Parmesan

Ingredients:
- 2 medium-sized zucchini
- 1/2 cup grated Parmesan cheese
- 1/2 cup breadcrumbs (you can use regular or panko breadcrumbs)

- 1 teaspoon garlic powder
- 1 teaspoon dried oregano
- 1/2 teaspoon salt
- 1/4 teaspoon black pepper
- 2 large eggs

Instructions:

- Preheat your oven to 425°F (220°C).
- Line a baking sheet with parchment paper or lightly grease it to prevent the zucchini chips from sticking.
- Wash the zucchini and slice them into thin rounds, about 1/8 to 1/4 inch thick.
- In a shallow bowl, combine the grated Parmesan cheese, breadcrumbs, garlic powder, dried oregano, salt, and black pepper. Mix well to evenly distribute the seasonings.
- In another bowl, whisk the eggs.
- Dip each zucchini slice into the whisked eggs, ensuring it's coated on both sides.
- After dipping in the eggs, transfer the zucchini slice to the Parmesan mixture. Coat it thoroughly with the mixture, pressing it on to adhere.
- Place the coated zucchini slices on the prepared baking sheet in a single layer, ensuring they are not touching.
- Bake in the preheated oven for about 15-20 minutes or until the zucchini chips are golden brown and crispy. Keep an eye on them to prevent burning.
- Once done, remove from the oven and let them cool for a few minutes before serving.
- You can serve the zucchini chips with a dipping sauce of your choice, such as marinara or ranch.

Edamame and Sea Salt Pods

Ingredients:

- 2 cups of frozen edamame pods
- 1 tablespoon sea salt (adjust to taste)

Instructions:

- Bring a large pot of water to a boil.
- Add a pinch of salt to the boiling water.
- Add the frozen edamame pods to the boiling water.
- Boil for about 4-5 minutes or until the edamame pods are tender.
- Once the edamame is done, drain them in a colander.
- Transfer the boiled edamame pods to a large mixing bowl.
- While the edamame pods are still warm, sprinkle them with sea salt.
- Toss the edamame pods in the bowl to ensure they are evenly coated with sea salt.
- Serve the edamame pods in a bowl or on a plate.

- Optionally, you can sprinkle a bit more sea salt on top for extra flavor.
- Edamame with sea salt is now ready to be enjoyed as a healthy and delicious snack!

Mango Chili Lime Salsa

Ingredients:
- 2 ripe mangoes, diced
- 1/2 red onion, finely chopped
- 1-2 jalapeños, seeded and finely chopped (adjust to taste)
- 1/4 cup fresh cilantro, chopped
- Juice of 2 limes
- Zest of 1 lime
- Salt and pepper to taste

Instructions:
- Peel and dice the ripe mangoes. If you're not familiar with how to cut a mango, you can find many tutorials online.
- Finely chop the red onion and jalapeños. Adjust the amount of jalapeños based on your spice preference.
- Chop the fresh cilantro. You can include both the leaves and the tender stems.
- In a bowl, combine the diced mangoes, chopped red onion, jalapeños, and cilantro.
- Squeeze the juice of 2 limes over the mixture. Also, add the zest of 1 lime for an extra burst of flavor.
- Season the salsa with salt and pepper to taste. Start with a small amount and adjust according to your preference.
- Gently toss all the ingredients together until well combined. Be careful not to mash the mangoes; you want to maintain some texture.
- Allow the salsa to chill in the refrigerator for at least 30 minutes before serving. This helps the flavors meld together.
- Once chilled, give the salsa a final stir and serve it with tortilla chips, grilled chicken, fish, or as a topping for tacos.

Walnut-Stuffed Celery

Ingredients:
- 1 bunch of celery
- 1 cup of cream cheese, softened
- 1 cup of chopped walnuts
- 2 tablespoons of chopped fresh parsley
- Salt and pepper to taste

Instructions:

- Wash the celery thoroughly and cut off the root end.
- Separate the celery stalks and trim them to your desired length, typically 4-6 inches.
- In a mixing bowl, combine the softened cream cheese, chopped walnuts, and chopped parsley.
- Season the mixture with salt and pepper to taste.
- Mix everything well until the ingredients are evenly distributed.
- Using a butter knife or a small spoon, carefully fill each celery stalk with the walnut and cream cheese mixture.
- Ensure that the filling is evenly distributed along the length of each celery stalk.
- Place the stuffed celery in the refrigerator for at least 30 minutes to allow the flavors to meld and the cream cheese to set slightly.
- Once chilled, arrange the stuffed celery on a serving platter and garnish with additional chopped parsley if desired.
- Serve the walnut-stuffed celery as an appetizer at parties, gatherings, or any occasion.
- Enjoy the delightful combination of crunchy celery and creamy walnut filling.

Chocolate-Dipped Strawberries

Ingredients:

- Fresh strawberries (1 pound or as desired)
- Dark or milk chocolate chips (8 ounces)
- White chocolate chips (optional, for drizzling)
- Toppings (optional, e.g., chopped nuts, shredded coconut, sprinkles)

Instructions:

Prepare the Strawberries:

- Wash and dry the strawberries thoroughly. It's important to start with dry strawberries so that the chocolate adheres well.

Melt the Chocolate:

- Place the dark or milk chocolate chips in a heatproof bowl. You can use a double boiler or microwave to melt the chocolate.
- If using a double boiler, melt the chocolate over simmering water, stirring until smooth.
- If using a microwave, heat the chocolate in 20-second intervals, stirring between each interval until fully melted.

Dip the Strawberries:

- Hold each strawberry by the stem and dip it into the melted chocolate, ensuring that the strawberry is fully coated.
- Allow any excess chocolate to drip off back into the bowl.

Set on Parchment Paper:
- Place the chocolate-dipped strawberries on a parchment paper-lined tray or plate. This will prevent them from sticking and make for easy cleanup.

Optional Toppings:
- While the chocolate is still wet, you can sprinkle or roll the dipped strawberries in toppings like chopped nuts, shredded coconut, or sprinkles for added flavor and texture.

Cool and Set:
- Allow the chocolate-dipped strawberries to cool and set. You can place them in the refrigerator for faster setting.

Drizzle with White Chocolate (Optional):
- If desired, melt the white chocolate chips using the same method as the dark or milk chocolate. Drizzle the melted white chocolate over the set dark chocolate-dipped strawberries for a decorative touch.

Final Setting:
- Allow the white chocolate drizzle to set, either at room temperature or in the refrigerator.

Serve:
- Once the chocolate is fully set, your chocolate-dipped strawberries are ready to be served! Arrange them on a plate and enjoy.

Tuna Salad Lettuce Wraps

Ingredients:
- 2 cans (about 10 ounces each) of tuna, drained
- 1/2 cup mayonnaise
- 1/4 cup diced red onion
- 1/4 cup diced celery
- 1 tablespoon Dijon mustard
- 1 tablespoon lemon juice
- Salt and pepper to taste
- Lettuce leaves (such as iceberg or butter lettuce) for wrapping

Instructions:
- In a mixing bowl, combine the drained tuna, mayonnaise, diced red onion, diced celery, Dijon mustard, and lemon juice.
- Mix the ingredients well until everything is evenly combined.
- Season the tuna salad with salt and pepper to taste. Adjust the seasoning according to your preferences.
- Wash and pat dry the lettuce leaves. These will be used as the wraps.
- Spoon the tuna salad mixture onto each lettuce leaf, distributing it evenly.
- Carefully fold or roll the lettuce leaves around the tuna salad, creating a wrap.
- Secure the wraps with toothpicks if needed.
- Serve immediately and enjoy your Tuna Salad Lettuce Wraps!

Curry Spiced Popcorn

Ingredients:

- 1/2 cup popcorn kernels
- 3 tablespoons vegetable oil
- 2 teaspoons curry powder
- 1 teaspoon ground cumin
- 1 teaspoon ground coriander
- 1/2 teaspoon turmeric
- 1/4 teaspoon cayenne pepper (adjust to taste)
- Salt to taste

Instructions:

Pop the Popcorn:

- In a large pot with a tight-fitting lid, heat the vegetable oil over medium heat.
- Add 2-3 popcorn kernels to the pot. Once they pop, the oil is hot enough.
- Add the remaining popcorn kernels, cover the pot with the lid, and shake it gently to coat the kernels with oil.
- Continue shaking occasionally to prevent burning. When the popping slows down, remove the pot from heat.

Prepare the Spice Mixture:

- In a small bowl, mix together the curry powder, ground cumin, ground coriander, turmeric, cayenne pepper, and salt. Adjust the spice levels according to your preference.

Combine Popcorn and Spices:

- Drizzle the spice mixture over the popped popcorn. You can do this in layers, adding spice and shaking to distribute evenly.

Toss and Serve:

- Toss the popcorn gently to ensure even coating of the spices.
- Taste and adjust the seasoning if necessary.

Optional Additions:

- For added flavor, you can sprinkle a bit of nutritional yeast or grated Parmesan cheese over the popcorn.

Serve and Enjoy:

- Transfer the spiced popcorn to a serving bowl and enjoy your curry-spiced popcorn!

Protein-Packed Chia Pudding

Ingredients:

- 1/4 cup chia seeds
- 1 cup milk (dairy or plant-based)
- 1 scoop protein powder (flavor of your choice)
- 1-2 tablespoons sweetener (such as honey, maple syrup, or agave nectar)
- 1/2 teaspoon vanilla extract

- Optional toppings: fresh fruits, nuts, seeds, or granola

Instructions:

Mixing the Base:

- In a bowl or jar, combine the chia seeds, milk, protein powder, sweetener, and vanilla extract.
- Whisk the ingredients together thoroughly to ensure that the chia seeds are well distributed and don't clump together.

Setting Time:

- Cover the bowl or jar and refrigerate the mixture for at least 3 hours or overnight. This allows the chia seeds to absorb the liquid and create a pudding-like consistency.

Stirring Occasionally:

- After the first hour, give the mixture a good stir to prevent clumping. Repeat this process at least once more before it's fully set.

Toppings:

- Once the chia pudding has reached the desired consistency, you can add your favorite toppings. Fresh fruits, nuts, seeds, or granola are great choices for added flavor, texture, and nutrition.

Serve and Enjoy:

- Scoop the chia pudding into a serving bowl or eat it directly from the jar. Customize with additional toppings as desired.

Flavorful Dinners for Diabetes Management

Grilled Lemon Herb Salmon

Ingredients:

- 4 salmon fillets (about 6 ounces each)
- 2 lemons (1 for juice, 1 for slices)
- 3 tablespoons olive oil
- 2 cloves garlic, minced
- 1 teaspoon dried thyme
- 1 teaspoon dried rosemary
- 1 teaspoon dried oregano
- Salt and pepper to taste
- Fresh parsley, chopped (for garnish)

Instructions:

- In a small bowl, whisk together the olive oil, minced garlic, dried thyme, dried rosemary, dried oregano, salt, and pepper.
- Squeeze the juice of one lemon into the mixture and whisk until well combined.
- Place the salmon fillets in a shallow dish or a large zip-top bag.
- Pour the marinade over the salmon, ensuring each fillet is well-coated.
- Cover the dish or seal the bag and let it marinate in the refrigerator for at least 30 minutes. You can marinate it longer for more flavor, even overnight.
- Preheat your grill to medium-high heat.
- Remove the salmon from the refrigerator and let it come to room temperature for about 10-15 minutes.
- Place the marinated salmon fillets on the preheated grill.
- Grill for about 4-5 minutes per side, or until the salmon is cooked to your liking. The internal temperature should reach 145°F (63°C).
- In the last couple of minutes of grilling, add lemon slices to the grill and cook them until they have grill marks.
- Transfer the grilled salmon to a serving platter.
- Squeeze the grilled lemon slices over the salmon for an extra burst of flavor.
- Garnish with fresh chopped parsley.
- Serve the grilled lemon herb salmon with your favorite sides, such as steamed vegetables, rice, or a fresh salad.

Mediterranean Chicken Skewers

Ingredients:

- 1.5 lbs (about 700g) boneless, skinless chicken breasts, cut into bite-sized cubes
- 1/4 cup olive oil

- 3 cloves garlic, minced
- 1 teaspoon dried oregano
- 1 teaspoon dried thyme
- 1 teaspoon paprika
- 1 teaspoon ground cumin
- Salt and black pepper to taste
- Zest and juice of 1 lemon
- 1 red bell pepper, cut into chunks
- 1 yellow bell pepper, cut into chunks
- 1 red onion, cut into chunks
- Cherry tomatoes (optional)
- Wooden skewers, soaked in water for at least 30 minutes

Instructions:

- In a bowl, mix together the olive oil, minced garlic, oregano, thyme, paprika, cumin, salt, black pepper, lemon zest, and lemon juice. This will be your marinade.
- Place the chicken cubes in a large zip-top bag or shallow dish and pour half of the marinade over them. Toss to coat the chicken evenly. Seal the bag or cover the dish and refrigerate for at least 30 minutes to marinate. You can also marinate it for several hours or overnight for more flavor.
- Preheat your grill or grill pan over medium-high heat.
- While the grill is heating, thread the marinated chicken, bell peppers, red onion, and cherry tomatoes (if using) onto the soaked wooden skewers, alternating the ingredients.
- Brush the skewers with the remaining marinade.
- Grill the skewers for about 8-10 minutes, turning occasionally, or until the chicken is fully cooked and has nice grill marks.
- Serve the Mediterranean Chicken Skewers with your favorite side dishes like couscous, rice, or a Greek salad.
- Enjoy your delicious Mediterranean Chicken Skewers!

Cauliflower Fried Rice with Shrimp

Ingredients:

- 1 medium-sized cauliflower
- 1 pound (about 450g) shrimp, peeled and deveined
- 2 tablespoons vegetable oil
- 1 cup mixed vegetables (carrots, peas, corn, diced bell peppers, etc.)
- 3 cloves garlic, minced
- 2 eggs, beaten
- 3 green onions, finely chopped
- 3 tablespoons soy sauce

- 1 tablespoon oyster sauce
- 1 teaspoon sesame oil
- Salt and pepper to taste
- Optional: Sriracha or chili sauce for added heat

Instructions:

Prepare the Cauliflower Rice:

- Cut the cauliflower into florets and place them in a food processor.
- Pulse until the cauliflower resembles rice-sized grains. Be careful not to over-process; you want a rice-like texture.
- Set aside the cauliflower rice.

Cook the Shrimp:

- Heat 1 tablespoon of vegetable oil in a large skillet or wok over medium-high heat.
- Add the shrimp and cook until they turn pink and opaque, about 2-3 minutes per side.
- Remove the shrimp from the pan and set aside.

Stir-Fry Vegetables:

- In the same pan, add another tablespoon of oil.
- Add minced garlic and stir-fry for about 30 seconds until fragrant.
- Add the mixed vegetables and cook until they are tender-crisp.

Add Cauliflower Rice:

- Push the vegetables to one side of the pan, and add the cauliflower rice to the empty space.
- Stir-fry the cauliflower rice for 3-4 minutes until it's cooked but still has a slight crunch.

Combine Ingredients:

- Mix the cauliflower rice with the vegetables in the pan.
- Push the mixture to the sides to create a well in the center.

Scramble Eggs:

- Pour the beaten eggs into the well and scramble them until they're fully cooked.

Add Shrimp and Sauce:

- Add the cooked shrimp back to the pan.
- Pour soy sauce, oyster sauce, and sesame oil over the mixture.
- Stir everything together until it is well combined.

Season and Garnish:

- Season with salt and pepper to taste.
- Stir in chopped green onions.
- Optional: Add a drizzle of Sriracha or your favorite chili sauce for extra heat.

Serve:

- Serve the cauliflower fried rice with shrimp hot, garnished with additional green onions if desired.
- Enjoy your delicious and low-carb cauliflower fried rice with shrimp!

Balsamic Glazed Turkey Meatballs

Ingredients:
- For the Meatballs:
- 1 pound ground turkey
- 1/2 cup breadcrumbs
- 1/4 cup grated Parmesan cheese
- 1/4 cup chopped fresh parsley
- 1 large egg
- 2 cloves garlic, minced
- Salt and pepper to taste
- Olive oil for cooking

For the Balsamic Glaze:
- 1/2 cup balsamic vinegar
- 1/4 cup honey
- 2 tablespoons soy sauce
- 1 teaspoon Dijon mustard

Instructions:
- Preheat your oven to 375°F (190°C).
- In a large mixing bowl, combine ground turkey, breadcrumbs, Parmesan cheese, chopped parsley, minced garlic, egg, salt, and pepper. Mix until well combined.
- Shape the mixture into small meatballs, about 1 inch in diameter, and place them on a baking sheet lined with parchment paper.
- Heat olive oil in a large skillet over medium heat. Add the meatballs and cook until browned on all sides, about 3-4 minutes.
- While the meatballs are cooking, prepare the balsamic glaze. In a small saucepan, combine balsamic vinegar, honey, soy sauce, and Dijon mustard. Bring the mixture to a simmer over medium heat and let it cook for 5-7 minutes, or until the glaze thickens.
- Transfer the browned meatballs to a baking dish and drizzle the balsamic glaze over them.
- Bake in the preheated oven for 15-20 minutes, or until the meatballs are cooked through.
- Optional: Garnish with additional chopped parsley and serve with your favorite side dishes.

Spaghetti Squash Primavera

Ingredients:
- 1 medium-sized spaghetti squash
- 2 tablespoons olive oil
- 3 cloves garlic, minced

- 1 small red onion, thinly sliced
- 1 bell pepper, thinly sliced (use a mix of colors for visual appeal)
- 1 zucchini, thinly sliced
- 1 yellow squash, thinly sliced
- 1 cup cherry tomatoes, halved
- 1/2 cup grated Parmesan cheese
- Salt and pepper, to taste
- Red pepper flakes (optional, for added spice)
- Fresh basil or parsley, chopped (for garnish)

Instructions:

- Preheat your oven to 400°F (200°C).
- Cut the spaghetti squash in half lengthwise and scoop out the seeds. Place the squash halves, cut side down, on a baking sheet. Roast in the preheated oven for about 40-45 minutes, or until the squash is tender.
- While the squash is roasting, heat olive oil in a large skillet over medium heat. Add minced garlic and sauté for about 1 minute until fragrant.
- Add sliced red onion to the skillet and sauté for 2-3 minutes until softened.
- Add the bell peppers, zucchini, and yellow squash to the skillet. Cook for another 5-7 minutes until the vegetables are tender-crisp.
- Stir in the cherry tomatoes and cook for an additional 2-3 minutes until they are just heated through.
- Once the spaghetti squash is done roasting, use a fork to scrape the flesh into strands.
- Add the spaghetti squash strands to the skillet with the sautéed vegetables. Toss everything together until well combined.
- Season the dish with salt, pepper, and red pepper flakes (if using). Adjust the seasoning according to your taste.
- Sprinkle grated Parmesan cheese over the top and toss until the cheese is melted and the vegetables are evenly coated.
- Garnish with fresh, chopped basil or parsley.
- Serve warm and enjoy your Spaghetti Squash Primavera!

Feel free to customize the recipe by adding your favorite vegetables or protein sources, like grilled chicken or shrimp.

Stuffed Bell Peppers with Quinoa and Black Beans

Ingredients:

- 4 large bell peppers (any color)
- 1 cup quinoa, rinsed
- 2 cups vegetable broth or water
- 1 can (15 oz) black beans, drained and rinsed

- 1 cup corn kernels (fresh or frozen)
- 1 cup diced tomatoes
- 1 cup shredded cheese (cheddar, Monterey Jack, or your choice)
- 1 small onion, finely chopped
- 2 cloves garlic, minced
- 1 teaspoon cumin
- 1 teaspoon chili powder
- Salt and pepper to taste
- Olive oil for cooking
- Fresh cilantro or parsley for garnish (optional)

Instructions:
- Preheat your oven to 375°F (190°C).
- In a medium saucepan, combine the quinoa and vegetable broth (or water). Bring to a boil, then reduce heat to low, cover, and simmer for about 15 minutes or until the quinoa is cooked and the liquid is absorbed.
- Cut the tops off the bell peppers and remove the seeds and membranes. Lightly brush the outside of the peppers with olive oil and place them in a baking dish.
- In a large skillet, heat olive oil over medium heat. Add the chopped onion and garlic, sautéing until softened.
- Add the black beans, corn, diced tomatoes, cumin, chili powder, salt, and pepper to the skillet. Cook for an additional 5-7 minutes until the mixture is heated through.
- Stir in the cooked quinoa and 1/2 cup of shredded cheese. Mix well until everything is combined.
- Spoon the quinoa and black bean mixture into each bell pepper until they are full. Press the filling down gently, and top each pepper with a sprinkle of the remaining shredded cheese.
- Cover the baking dish with foil and bake in the preheated oven for 25-30 minutes, or until the peppers are tender.
- Remove from the oven and let them cool for a few minutes before serving. Garnish with fresh cilantro or parsley, if desired.

Teriyaki Tofu Stir-Fry

Ingredients:
- 1 block of firm tofu, pressed and cubed
- 2 cups broccoli florets
- 1 bell pepper, thinly sliced
- 1 carrot, julienned
- 1 cup snow peas, ends trimmed
- 1 tablespoon vegetable oil

For the Teriyaki Sauce:

- 1/4 cup soy sauce
- 2 tablespoons water
- 2 tablespoons rice vinegar
- 2 tablespoons brown sugar
- 1 tablespoon mirin (Japanese sweet rice wine)
- 1 teaspoon sesame oil
- 2 cloves garlic, minced
- 1 teaspoon grated ginger
- 1 tablespoon cornstarch (for thickening)

Optional toppings:

- Sesame seeds
- Green onions, chopped
- Cooked rice or noodles for serving

Instructions:

Prepare the Tofu:

- Press the tofu to remove excess water. Cut it into cubes.
- Heat 1 tablespoon of vegetable oil in a large skillet or wok over medium-high heat.
- Add tofu cubes and cook until all sides are golden brown. Remove tofu from the pan and set aside.

Prepare the Vegetables:

- In the same pan, add a little more oil if needed.
- Stir-fry broccoli, bell pepper, carrot, and snow peas until they are crisp-tender.

Make the Teriyaki Sauce:

- In a small bowl, whisk together the soy sauce, water, rice vinegar, brown sugar, mirin, sesame oil, minced garlic, and grated ginger.
- In a separate small bowl, mix the cornstarch with a little water to create a slurry.

Combine and Cook:

- Pour the teriyaki sauce over the stir-fried vegetables.
- Add the cooked tofu back to the pan and toss everything together.
- Pour the cornstarch slurry into the pan to thicken the sauce. Stir well to coat everything evenly.

Serve:

- Once the sauce has thickened, remove the pan from heat.
- Serve the Teriyaki Tofu Stir-Fry over cooked rice or noodles.
- Garnish with sesame seeds and chopped green onions, if desired.

Lemon Garlic Herb Grilled Chicken

Ingredients:

- 4 boneless, skinless chicken breasts
- 1/4 cup olive oil
- 3 cloves garlic, minced
- Zest and juice of 1 lemon
- 1 teaspoon dried oregano
- 1 teaspoon dried thyme
- 1 teaspoon dried rosemary
- Salt and pepper to taste

Instructions:

- In a small bowl, whisk together the olive oil, minced garlic, lemon zest, lemon juice, oregano, thyme, rosemary, salt, and pepper. This will be your marinade.
- Place the chicken breasts in a resealable plastic bag or a shallow dish.
- Pour the marinade over the chicken, making sure each piece is well-coated. Seal the bag or cover the dish, and let it marinate in the refrigerator for at least 30 minutes to allow the flavors to penetrate the chicken.
- Preheat your grill to medium-high heat.
- Remove the chicken from the marinade, allowing any excess to drip off.
- Place the chicken on the preheated grill and cook for about 6-8 minutes per side, or until the internal temperature reaches 165°F (74°C) and the chicken is no longer pink in the center.
- Baste the chicken with any remaining marinade during grilling to keep it moist and flavorful.
- Once cooked, remove the chicken from the grill and let it rest for a few minutes before serving.
- Serve the Lemon Garlic Herb Grilled Chicken with your favorite side dishes and enjoy!

Zucchini Noodles with Pesto and Cherry Tomatoes

Ingredients:

- 4 medium-sized zucchini
- 1 cup cherry tomatoes, halved
- 1/2 cup basil pesto (homemade or store-bought)
- 2 tablespoons olive oil
- Salt and pepper to taste
- Grated Parmesan cheese for garnish (optional)

Instructions:

- Using a spiralizer or a vegetable peeler, create zucchini noodles. If using a peeler, make wide ribbons by dragging it along the length of the zucchini.
- If you prefer, you can lightly salt the zucchini noodles and let them sit in a colander for about 15 minutes to release excess moisture. Then, pat them dry with paper towels.
- Heat olive oil in a large skillet over medium heat.
- Add the zucchini noodles and sauté for 2-3 minutes until just tender. Be careful not to overcook; you want the noodles to retain some crunch.
- Toss in the halved cherry tomatoes and cook for an additional 1-2 minutes until they start to soften.
- Reduce heat to low and add the basil pesto to the skillet, tossing the zucchini noodles and tomatoes until evenly coated.
- Season with salt and pepper to taste. Remember that the pesto and Parmesan (if using) already contribute to the overall saltiness.
- Once everything is heated through, remove from heat.
- Optionally, garnish with grated Parmesan cheese and additional fresh basil.
- Serve immediately, and enjoy your healthy and delicious zucchini noodles with pesto and cherry tomatoes!

Indian-Spiced Lentil Curry

Ingredients:

- 1 cup dry lentils (red or brown), rinsed and drained
- 2 tablespoons vegetable oil
- 1 large onion, finely chopped
- 3 cloves garlic, minced
- 1 tablespoon ginger, grated
- 1 can (14 oz) diced tomatoes
- 1 can (14 oz) coconut milk
- 1 cup vegetable broth or water
- 2 teaspoons curry powder
- 1 teaspoon ground cumin
- 1 teaspoon ground coriander
- 1/2 teaspoon turmeric
- 1/2 teaspoon cayenne pepper (adjust to taste)
- Salt and pepper to taste
- Fresh cilantro, chopped (for garnish)
- Cooked rice or naan bread (for serving)

Instructions:

Prepare Lentils:

- Rinse the lentils under cold water until the water runs clear.

- In a medium-sized pot, combine the lentils with enough water to cover them by about an inch. Bring to a boil, then reduce heat and simmer until lentils are tender but not mushy (about 15-20 minutes). Drain any excess water.

Sauté Aromatics:
- In a large skillet or pot, heat the vegetable oil over medium heat.
- Add chopped onions and cook until they become translucent.

Add Garlic and Ginger:
- Stir in minced garlic and grated ginger, and cook for another 1-2 minutes until fragrant.

Spices:
- Add curry powder, ground cumin, ground coriander, turmeric, and cayenne pepper. Stir well to coat the onions and aromatics with the spices.

Tomatoes:
- Pour in the diced tomatoes with their juices. Cook for 5-7 minutes until the tomatoes break down and the mixture thickens.

Coconut Milk and Broth:
- Stir in the coconut milk and vegetable broth (or water). Bring the mixture to a simmer.

Combine Lentils:
- Add the cooked lentils to the pot, stirring well to combine. Allow it to simmer for an additional 10-15 minutes, allowing the flavors to meld.

Seasoning:
- Season the curry with salt and pepper to taste. Adjust the spice level if needed.

Serve:
- Serve the lentil curry over cooked rice or with naan bread.
- Garnish with fresh cilantro.

Salmon and Asparagus Foil Packets

Ingredients:
- 4 salmon fillets
- 1 bunch of asparagus, trimmed
- 1 lemon, thinly sliced
- 4 cloves of garlic, minced
- 4 tablespoons olive oil
- Salt and pepper to taste
- Fresh herbs (such as dill, parsley, or thyme) for garnish
- Optional: 1 tablespoon honey or Dijon mustard for extra flavor

Instructions:
- Preheat your oven to 400°F (200°C).
- Cut four large pieces of aluminum foil, each about 12 inches long.
- Place a salmon fillet in the center of each piece of foil.
- Drizzle each salmon fillet with 1 tablespoon of olive oil.

- Sprinkle minced garlic over the salmon.
- Season with salt and pepper to taste.
- Optionally, drizzle with honey or spread a bit of Dijon mustard for extra flavor.
- Arrange a handful of trimmed asparagus next to each salmon fillet.
- Place a couple of lemon slices on top of each fillet.
- Fold the sides of the foil over the salmon and asparagus, creating a packet.
- Seal the edges tightly to prevent any juices from leaking.
- Place the foil packets on a baking sheet and bake in the preheated oven for about 15-20 minutes, or until the salmon is cooked through and flakes easily with a fork.
- Carefully open the foil packets (watch out for steam) and garnish with fresh herbs.
- Serve the salmon and asparagus directly from the foil packets or transfer to plates.

Cajun Shrimp and Sausage Skillet

Ingredients:
- 1 pound large shrimp, peeled and deveined
- 1 pound Andouille sausage, sliced
- 1 bell pepper, diced
- 1 onion, diced
- 3 cloves garlic, minced
- 1 can (14 ounces) diced tomatoes, undrained
- 1 teaspoon Cajun seasoning (adjust to taste)
- 1/2 teaspoon dried thyme
- 1/2 teaspoon dried oregano
- 1/4 teaspoon cayenne pepper (optional, for extra heat)
- Salt and black pepper to taste
- 2 tablespoons olive oil
- Fresh parsley, chopped (for garnish)
- Cooked rice, for serving

Instructions:
Prepare Ingredients:
- Clean and devein the shrimp.
- Slice the Andouille sausage.
- Dice the bell pepper and onion.
- Mince the garlic.

Season Shrimp:
- In a bowl, season the shrimp with Cajun seasoning. Set aside.

Sauté Sausage:
- Heat olive oil in a large skillet over medium heat.
- Add the sliced Andouille sausage and cook until browned on both sides.

Add Vegetables:

- Add diced onion, bell pepper, and minced garlic to the skillet. Sauté until vegetables are softened.

Spices and Tomatoes:

- Stir in Cajun seasoning, dried thyme, dried oregano, and cayenne pepper (if using).
- Pour in diced tomatoes with their juices. Stir well to combine.

Cook Shrimp:

- Add seasoned shrimp to the skillet and cook until they turn pink and opaque.

Adjust Seasoning:

- Taste the mixture and adjust the seasoning with salt and black pepper, as needed.

Serve:

- Serve the Cajun shrimp and sausage over cooked rice.

Garnish:

- Garnish with chopped fresh parsley before serving.

Roasted Vegetable and Chickpea Salad

Ingredients:

- 2 cups cherry tomatoes, halved
- 1 large red bell pepper, sliced
- 1 large yellow bell pepper, sliced
- 1 medium zucchini, sliced
- 1 medium red onion, thinly sliced
- 1 can (15 oz) chickpeas, drained and rinsed
- 3 tablespoons olive oil
- 1 teaspoon dried oregano
- 1 teaspoon dried thyme
- Salt and black pepper, to taste
- 4 cups mixed salad greens (e.g., arugula, spinach, or your choice)
- 1/4 cup feta cheese, crumbled (optional)

For the dressing:

- 3 tablespoons extra-virgin olive oil
- 2 tablespoons balsamic vinegar
- 1 teaspoon Dijon mustard
- Salt and black pepper, to taste

Instructions:

- Preheat your oven to 400°F (200°C).
- In a large mixing bowl, combine the cherry tomatoes, red bell pepper, yellow bell pepper, zucchini, red onion, and chickpeas.

- Drizzle the vegetables and chickpeas with 3 tablespoons of olive oil. Sprinkle with dried oregano, dried thyme, salt, and black pepper. Toss everything together until the vegetables and chickpeas are well coated with the oil and seasonings.
- Spread the vegetable and chickpea mixture evenly on a baking sheet lined with parchment paper.
- Roast in the preheated oven for 25-30 minutes or until the vegetables are tender and slightly caramelized, stirring halfway through.
- While the vegetables are roasting, prepare the dressing. In a small bowl, whisk together the extra-virgin olive oil, balsamic vinegar, Dijon mustard, salt, and black pepper. Set aside.
- Once the roasted vegetables and chickpeas are done, remove them from the oven and let them cool slightly.
- In a large salad bowl, combine the roasted vegetables and chickpeas with the mixed salad greens.
- Drizzle the salad with the prepared dressing and toss everything together until well combined.
- If desired, sprinkle crumbled feta cheese over the top.
- Serve immediately and enjoy your delicious Roasted Vegetable and Chickpea Salad!

Turkey and Vegetable Lettuce Wraps

Ingredients:
- 1 lb ground turkey
- 1 tablespoon olive oil
- 1 onion, finely chopped
- 2 cloves garlic, minced
- 1 red bell pepper, diced
- 1 zucchini, diced
- 1 carrot, julienned or shredded
- 1 cup mushrooms, chopped
- 1 teaspoon ground cumin
- 1 teaspoon chili powder
- Salt and pepper to taste
- 1/4 cup soy sauce or tamari for a gluten-free option
- 1 tablespoon hoisin sauce
- 1 tablespoon rice vinegar
- 1 tablespoon sesame oil
- 1 head iceberg or butter lettuce, leaves separated

Instructions:

- Heat olive oil in a large skillet over medium heat.
- Add chopped onion and minced garlic to the skillet and sauté until softened.
- Add ground turkey to the skillet, breaking it apart with a spatula, and cook until browned.
- Stir in diced red bell pepper, zucchini, shredded carrot, and chopped mushrooms. Cook for an additional 3-5 minutes until the vegetables are tender.
- Season the mixture with ground cumin, chili powder, salt, and pepper. Stir well to combine.
- In a small bowl, whisk together soy sauce (or tamari), hoisin sauce, rice vinegar, and sesame oil. Pour the sauce over the turkey and vegetable mixture, stirring to coat evenly. Cook for an additional 2-3 minutes.
- Remove the skillet from heat and let the mixture cool slightly.
- To serve, spoon the turkey and vegetable mixture into individual lettuce leaves, creating wraps.
- Optionally, you can garnish with chopped green onions, cilantro, or sesame seeds.

Greek Chicken Souvlaki Bowl

Ingredients:

- 1 lb (450 g) boneless, skinless chicken breasts, cut into bite-sized pieces
- 2 tablespoons olive oil
- 2 tablespoons lemon juice
- 2 teaspoons dried oregano
- 1 teaspoon dried thyme
- 3 cloves garlic, minced
- Salt and pepper to taste

For the Tzatziki Sauce:

- 1 cup Greek yogurt
- 1 cucumber, grated
- 2 cloves garlic, minced
- 1 tablespoon fresh dill, chopped
- 1 tablespoon olive oil
- Salt and pepper to taste

For the Bowl:

- Cooked quinoa or rice
- Cherry tomatoes, halved
- Cucumber, sliced
- Red onion, thinly sliced
- Kalamata olives, pitted and sliced

- Feta cheese, crumbled

Instructions:
- In a bowl, combine olive oil, lemon juice, oregano, thyme, minced garlic, salt, and pepper. Add the chicken pieces to the marinade, making sure they are well coated. Cover and refrigerate for at least 30 minutes or overnight.
- Preheat the grill or grill pan over medium-high heat. Thread the marinated chicken pieces onto skewers.
- Grill the chicken skewers for 6-8 minutes, turning occasionally, until the chicken is fully cooked and has a nice char.
- While the chicken is cooking, prepare the tzatziki sauce. In a bowl, combine Greek yogurt, grated cucumber, minced garlic, chopped dill, olive oil, salt, and pepper. Mix well and refrigerate until ready to use.
- Assemble the bowls by placing a serving of cooked quinoa or rice at the bottom. Top with grilled chicken skewers, cherry tomatoes, cucumber slices, red onion slices, Kalamata olives, and crumbled feta cheese.
- Drizzle tzatziki sauce over the top of the bowl or serve it on the side.
- Garnish with additional fresh herbs, lemon wedges, or extra feta cheese if desired.
- Serve immediately and enjoy your delicious Greek Chicken Souvlaki Bowl!

Cabbage and Beef Stir-Fry

Ingredients:
- 1 pound (450g) beef sirloin or flank steak, thinly sliced
- 1 small cabbage, shredded
- 1 carrot, julienned
- 1 bell pepper, thinly sliced
- 3 cloves garlic, minced
- 1 tablespoon ginger, minced
- 3 tablespoons soy sauce
- 1 tablespoon oyster sauce
- 1 tablespoon sesame oil
- 1 tablespoon cornstarch
- 2 tablespoons vegetable oil (for cooking)
- Salt and pepper to taste
- Green onions, chopped (for garnish)
- Sesame seeds (optional, for garnish)

Instructions:
- In a bowl, mix the thinly sliced beef with soy sauce, oyster sauce, sesame oil, and cornstarch. Allow it to marinate for at least 15-20 minutes.

- Heat 1 tablespoon of vegetable oil in a large wok or skillet over medium-high heat.
- Add the marinated beef to the hot wok and stir-fry for 2-3 minutes or until the beef is browned and cooked through. Remove the beef from the wok and set it aside.
- In the same wok, add another tablespoon of vegetable oil. Stir in the minced garlic and ginger, and sauté for about 30 seconds until fragrant.
- Add the shredded cabbage, julienned carrot, and sliced bell pepper to the wok. Stir-fry the vegetables for 4-5 minutes or until they are tender-crisp.
- Return the cooked beef to the wok with the vegetables. Toss everything together until well combined and heated through.
- Season with salt and pepper, to taste. Adjust the seasoning if needed.
- Garnish with chopped green onions and sesame seeds, if desired.
- Serve the cabbage and beef stir-fry over rice or noodles.

Pesto Zoodle Bowl with Grilled Chicken

Ingredients:
- 2 medium-sized zucchinis (spiralized into zoodles)
- 2 boneless, skinless chicken breasts
- Salt and black pepper to taste
- 1 tablespoon olive oil

For the Pesto Sauce:
- 2 cups fresh basil leaves, packed
- 1/2 cup grated Parmesan cheese
- 1/2 cup pine nuts
- 3 cloves garlic, peeled
- 1/2 cup extra-virgin olive oil
- Salt and black pepper to taste
- Juice of half a lemon

Optional Garnish:
- Cherry tomatoes, halved
- Extra Parmesan cheese
- Fresh basil leaves

Instructions:
Prepare the Pesto Sauce:
- In a food processor, combine the basil, Parmesan cheese, pine nuts, and garlic.
- Pulse until coarsely chopped.
- With the food processor running, slowly pour in the olive oil until the mixture is well combined and smooth.

- Season with salt and pepper to taste, and add the lemon juice. Blend again until everything is incorporated.

Grill the Chicken:
- Preheat the grill or grill pan over medium-high heat.
- Season the chicken breasts with salt and pepper.
- Grill the chicken for about 6-8 minutes per side or until cooked through.
- Let the chicken rest for a few minutes before slicing it into strips.

Prepare the Zoodles:
- Spiralize the zucchinis into noodles using a spiralizer.
- Heat 1 tablespoon of olive oil in a large skillet over medium heat.
- Add the zoodles and sauté for 2-3 minutes or until just tender. Be careful not to overcook; you want them to retain a slight crunch.

Assemble the Bowl:
- Divide the zoodles among serving bowls.
- Top the zoodles with grilled chicken strips.
- Drizzle the pesto sauce over the chicken and zoodles.

Garnish and Serve:
- Garnish with halved cherry tomatoes, extra Parmesan cheese, and fresh basil leaves if desired.
- Serve immediately and enjoy your Pesto Zoodle Bowl with Grilled Chicken!

Baked Co with Mediterranean Salsa

Ingredients:

For Baked Cod:
- 4 cod fillets
- 2 tablespoons olive oil
- 2 cloves garlic, minced
- 1 teaspoon dried oregano
- 1 teaspoon dried thyme
- Salt and pepper to taste
- Lemon wedges for serving

For Mediterranean Salsa:
- 1 cup cherry tomatoes, halved
- 1/2 cucumber, diced
- 1/4 cup red onion, finely chopped
- 1/4 cup Kalamata olives, chopped
- 2 tablespoons fresh parsley, chopped
- 2 tablespoons feta cheese, crumbled
- 1 tablespoon extra virgin olive oil

- 1 tablespoon balsamic vinegar
- Salt and pepper to taste

Instructions:
- Preheat your oven to 400°F (200°C).
- In a small bowl, mix together olive oil, minced garlic, dried oregano, dried thyme, salt, and pepper.
- Place the cod fillets on a baking sheet lined with parchment paper or lightly greased.
- Brush the cod fillets with the olive oil mixture, ensuring they are well-coated.
- Bake the cod in the preheated oven for about 15-20 minutes or until the fish is cooked through and easily flakes with a fork.
- While the cod is baking, prepare the Mediterranean Salsa. In a medium bowl, combine cherry tomatoes, cucumber, red onion, Kalamata olives, parsley, and feta cheese.
- In a small bowl, whisk together extra virgin olive oil, balsamic vinegar, salt, and pepper. Pour this dressing over the salsa ingredients and toss gently to combine.
- Once the cod is done baking, remove it from the oven and serve it with a generous spoonful of Mediterranean Salsa on top.
- Garnish with additional fresh parsley, and serve with lemon wedges on the side.

Butter Herb Roasted Vegetables with Chicken

Ingredients:
- 4 boneless, skinless chicken breasts
- 1 pound baby potatoes, halved
- 1 pound baby carrots
- 1 pound Brussels sprouts, trimmed and halved
- 1 red bell pepper, sliced
- 1 yellow bell pepper, sliced
- 1/2 cup unsalted butter, melted
- 4 cloves garlic, minced
- 1 tablespoon fresh rosemary, chopped
- 1 tablespoon fresh thyme leaves
- Salt and black pepper, to taste
- Olive oil for drizzling

Instructions:
- Preheat your oven to 400°F (200°C).
- In a small bowl, mix together the melted butter, minced garlic, chopped rosemary, and thyme. Set aside.
- Place the chicken breasts in the center of a large baking sheet. Surround them with the halved baby potatoes, baby carrots, Brussels sprouts, and sliced bell peppers.

- Drizzle the vegetables with olive oil and season everything with salt and black pepper.
- Pour the butter and herb mixture evenly over the chicken and vegetables, making sure everything is coated.
- Toss the vegetables gently to ensure they are well coated in the butter and herb mixture.
- Roast in the preheated oven for about 25-30 minutes or until the chicken is cooked through (internal temperature reaches 165°F or 74°C) and the vegetables are tender and golden brown.
- Halfway through the cooking time, you can turn the chicken breasts and toss the vegetables for even cooking.
- Once done, remove from the oven and let it rest for a few minutes before serving.
- Serve the Butter Herb Roasted Vegetables with Chicken hot, garnished with additional fresh herbs if desired.

Cauliflower Mash with Garlic and Herbs

Ingredients:

- 1 large head of cauliflower, chopped into florets
- 3 cloves of garlic, minced
- 2 tablespoons olive oil
- 1/4 cup fresh herbs (such as parsley, thyme, or chives), chopped
- Salt and pepper to taste
- 1/4 cup grated Parmesan cheese (optional)

Instructions:

- Rinse the cauliflower florets under cold water.
- Steam or boil the cauliflower until very tender. This usually takes about 10-15 minutes.
- In a small pan, heat the olive oil over medium heat.
- Add minced garlic and sauté for 1-2 minutes until fragrant. Be careful not to burn the garlic.
- Once the cauliflower is tender, drain any excess water and transfer it to a large bowl.
- Use a potato masher or an immersion blender to mash the cauliflower until it reaches a smooth consistency. You can also use a food processor.
- Add the sautéed garlic and chopped herbs to the mashed cauliflower.
- Mix well to distribute the flavors evenly.
- Season the cauliflower mash with salt and pepper to taste. Adjust the seasoning according to your preferences.
- If you like, mix in grated Parmesan cheese for added richness. This step is optional.
- Transfer the cauliflower mash to a serving dish and garnish with additional herbs if desired.
- Serve the cauliflower mash as a delicious and healthy alternative to mashed potatoes. It pairs well with various dishes, and the garlic and herbs add a wonderful depth of flavor.

Roasted Brussels Sprouts with Balsamic Glaze

Ingredients:

- 1 lb Brussels sprouts, trimmed and halved
- 2 tablespoons olive oil
- Salt and black pepper to taste
- 1/4 cup balsamic vinegar
- 1 tablespoon honey or maple syrup (optional, for sweetness)
- 1-2 cloves garlic, minced (optional, for extra flavor)
- Parmesan cheese, grated (optional, for garnish)

Instructions:

- Preheat your oven to 400°F (200°C).
- Trim the ends of the Brussels sprouts and cut them in half. Remove any outer leaves that may be wilted or discolored.
- Place the halved Brussels sprouts in a large mixing bowl. Drizzle olive oil over them, and season with salt and black pepper. Toss well to ensure the Brussels sprouts are evenly coated.
- Spread the seasoned Brussels sprouts in a single layer on a baking sheet. Roast in the preheated oven for 20-25 minutes or until they are golden brown and crispy on the edges. You may want to toss them halfway through the cooking time for even roasting.
- While the Brussels sprouts are roasting, prepare the balsamic glaze. In a small saucepan, combine balsamic vinegar and honey (or maple syrup) over medium heat. Add minced garlic if using. Bring the mixture to a simmer and let it cook for 5-7 minutes or until it has reduced by half and has a syrupy consistency.
- Once the Brussels sprouts are done roasting, transfer them to a serving bowl. Drizzle the balsamic glaze over the roasted Brussels sprouts and toss gently to coat them evenly.
- Garnish with grated Parmesan cheese if desired. Serve the roasted Brussels sprouts with balsamic glaze immediately.

Zucchini Noodles with Pesto Sauce

Ingredients:

- For Zucchini Noodles:
- 4 medium-sized zucchini
- 2 tablespoons olive oil
- Salt and pepper to taste
- For Pesto Sauce:
- 2 cups fresh basil leaves, packed
- 1/2 cup grated Parmesan cheese
- 1/2 cup pine nuts or walnuts
- 3 cloves garlic, peeled
- 1/2 cup extra-virgin olive oil
- Salt and pepper to taste
- Optional: 1/2 cup grated Pecorino Romano cheese

Instructions:

Zucchini Noodles:

- Prepare Zucchini: Wash and trim the ends of the zucchini. Use a spiralizer to create zucchini noodles. If you don't have a spiralizer, you can use a vegetable peeler to make long, thin strips.
-

- Cook Zucchini Noodles: Heat 2 tablespoons of olive oil in a large pan over medium heat. Add the zucchini noodles and sauté for 2-3 minutes, tossing them gently with tongs. Cook just until they are slightly softened but still have a bit of crunch. Season with salt and pepper to taste.
- Drain Excess Moisture: Zucchini noodles release water as they cook. After sautéing, place the noodles in a colander to drain excess moisture.

Pesto Sauce:
- Combine Ingredients: In a food processor, combine the basil, Parmesan cheese, pine nuts or walnuts, and garlic. Pulse until the ingredients are finely chopped.
- Add Olive Oil: With the food processor running, slowly stream in the olive oil until the mixture is well combined and forms a smooth paste. Stop to scrape down the sides of the processor if needed.
- Season and Optional Cheese: Add salt and pepper to taste. If you like, you can also stir in the optional Pecorino Romano cheese for an extra layer of flavor.

Assemble:
- Mix Pesto and Zucchini Noodles: In the pan with the cooked zucchini noodles, add the desired amount of pesto sauce. Toss the noodles until they are evenly coated with the pesto.
- Serve: Plate the zucchini noodles and, if desired, garnish with additional Parmesan cheese or fresh basil leaves. Serve immediately.

Enjoy your healthy and delicious Zucchini Noodles with Pesto Sauce!

Green Bean Almondine with Lemon Zest

Ingredients:
- 1 pound fresh green beans, trimmed
- 1/2 cup sliced almonds
- 2 tablespoons unsalted butter
- 1 tablespoon olive oil
- 2 cloves garlic, minced
- Zest of 1 lemon
- Salt and pepper, to taste
- Lemon wedges for serving (optional)

Instructions:
Blanch the Green Beans:
- Bring a large pot of salted water to a boil.
- Add the green beans and cook for 2-3 minutes, or until they are bright green and slightly tender but still crisp.

- Drain the green beans and immediately transfer them to a bowl of ice water to stop the cooking process.
- Once cooled, drain again and set aside.

Toast the Almonds:

- In a large skillet, heat the sliced almonds over medium heat.
- Toast the almonds, stirring frequently, until they are golden brown and fragrant. Be careful not to burn them.
- Remove the almonds from the skillet and set them aside.

Cook the Green Beans:

- In the same skillet, add the butter and olive oil over medium heat.
- Add the minced garlic and sauté for about 1 minute until fragrant.
- Add the blanched green beans to the skillet and toss to coat them in the butter and garlic mixture.
- Cook the green beans for 2-3 minutes, or until they are heated through and slightly caramelized.

Finish the Dish:

- Sprinkle the toasted almonds over the green beans and toss to combine.
- Add the lemon zest and toss again to distribute the flavors evenly.
- Season with salt and pepper, to taste.

Serve:

- Transfer the green beans and almonds to a serving platter.
- Garnish with additional lemon zest, if desired.
- Serve warm, with optional lemon wedges on the side for added freshness.

Spicy Roasted Broccoli with Parmesan

Ingredients:

- 1 pound (about 450g) fresh broccoli, washed and cut into florets
- 3 tablespoons olive oil
- 2 cloves garlic, minced
- 1 teaspoon crushed red pepper flakes (adjust to taste for spice level)
- Salt and black pepper to taste
- 1/2 cup (about 50g) grated Parmesan cheese
- Lemon wedges for serving (optional)

Instructions:

- Preheat your oven to 425°F (220°C).
- In a large mixing bowl, combine the broccoli florets, olive oil, minced garlic, crushed red pepper flakes, salt, and black pepper. Toss the ingredients until the broccoli is well coated.

- Spread the seasoned broccoli in a single layer on a baking sheet lined with parchment paper or aluminum foil.
- Roast the broccoli in the preheated oven for about 20-25 minutes or until the edges are crispy and golden brown. Be sure to toss the broccoli halfway through the cooking time to ensure even roasting.
- Once the broccoli is done, remove it from the oven and sprinkle the grated Parmesan cheese over the top. Return the baking sheet to the oven for an additional 2-3 minutes, or until the cheese is melted and bubbly.
- Carefully transfer the roasted broccoli to a serving dish, squeezing a bit of lemon juice over the top if desired.
- Serve the Spicy Roasted Broccoli with Parmesan as a side dish or snack. Enjoy!

Cabbage and Carrot Slaw with Apple Cider Vinaigrette

Ingredients:

For the slaw:
- 1/2 small head of green cabbage, thinly sliced or shredded
- 2 large carrots, grated
- 1/4 cup fresh parsley, chopped (optional, for garnish)

For the vinaigrette:
- 1/4 cup apple cider vinegar
- 2 tablespoons Dijon mustard
- 2 tablespoons honey or maple syrup
- 1/4 cup extra-virgin olive oil
- Salt and pepper to taste

Instructions:

Prepare the Vegetables:
- Thinly slice or shred the green cabbage.
- Grate the carrots using a box grater or food processor.
- If using, chop the fresh parsley.

Make the Vinaigrette:
- In a small bowl, whisk together apple cider vinegar, Dijon mustard, honey or maple syrup, and a pinch of salt and pepper.
- While whisking, slowly drizzle in the olive oil until the vinaigrette is well combined. Adjust the seasoning to taste.

Combine Slaw and Vinaigrette:
- In a large bowl, combine the sliced cabbage and grated carrots.
- Pour the apple cider vinaigrette over the vegetables.

Toss and Refrigerate:
- Toss the slaw and vinaigrette together until the vegetables are well coated.
- Cover the bowl and refrigerate for at least 30 minutes to allow the flavors to meld.

Serve:
- Before serving, toss the slaw again to ensure the dressing is evenly distributed.
- Garnish with fresh, chopped parsley if desired.

Mushroom and Spinach Stuffed Bell Peppers

Ingredients:
- 4 large bell peppers, halved and seeds removed
- 2 tablespoons olive oil
- 1 onion, finely chopped
- 2 cloves garlic, minced
- 8 ounces mushrooms, finely chopped
- 2 cups fresh spinach, chopped
- 1 cup cooked quinoa or rice
- 1 cup shredded mozzarella or your favorite cheese
- Salt and pepper to taste
- 1 teaspoon dried oregano
- 1 teaspoon dried basil
- 1/2 teaspoon red pepper flakes (optional)
- 1 can (14 ounces) diced tomatoes, drained
- Fresh parsley, chopped (for garnish)

Instructions:
- Preheat the Oven: Preheat your oven to 375°F (190°C).
- Prepare the Bell Peppers: Cut the bell peppers in half lengthwise, removing seeds and membranes. Place them in a baking dish.
- Sauté Onion and Garlic: In a large skillet, heat olive oil over medium heat. Add chopped onions and garlic and sauté until softened.
- Cook Mushrooms and Spinach: Add the finely chopped mushrooms to the skillet and cook until they release their moisture and become golden brown. Add the chopped spinach and cook until wilted. Season with salt and pepper.
- Combine with Quinoa (or Rice): Stir in the cooked quinoa or rice, dried oregano, dried basil, and red pepper flakes (if using). Mix well.
- Add Cheese: Remove the skillet from heat and stir in the shredded mozzarella or your favorite cheese until melted and well combined.
- Stuff the Peppers: Spoon the mushroom and spinach mixture into each halved bell pepper, pressing down gently to pack the filling.
- Top with Tomatoes: Top each stuffed pepper with diced tomatoes.

- Bake: Cover the baking dish with aluminum foil and bake in the preheated oven for 25-30 minutes or until the peppers are tender.
- Garnish and Serve: Remove from the oven, garnish with fresh chopped parsley, and serve hot.

Turmeric Roasted Sweet Potatoes

Ingredients:
- 3 large sweet potatoes, peeled and cut into 1-inch cubes
- 2 tablespoons olive oil
- 1 teaspoon ground turmeric
- 1 teaspoon ground cumin
- 1 teaspoon paprika
- 1/2 teaspoon garlic powder
- 1/2 teaspoon onion powder
- Salt and black pepper to taste
- Fresh parsley, chopped (for garnish, optional)

Instructions:
- Preheat your oven to 400°F (200°C).
- Peel the sweet potatoes and cut them into 1-inch cubes.
- In a small bowl, mix together the ground turmeric, cumin, paprika, garlic powder, onion powder, salt, and black pepper. Adjust the seasoning to your taste.
- Place the sweet potato cubes in a large bowl. Drizzle olive oil over the sweet potatoes and toss them until evenly coated.
- Sprinkle the spice mixture over the sweet potatoes. Toss again to ensure that the sweet potatoes are evenly coated with the spices.
- Spread the seasoned sweet potato cubes in a single layer on a baking sheet lined with parchment paper. Make sure they are not overcrowded to allow even roasting.
- Roast in the preheated oven for about 25-30 minutes or until the sweet potatoes are tender and golden brown. Remember to flip the sweet potatoes halfway through the cooking time for even roasting.
- Once done, remove from the oven and let them cool for a few minutes. Garnish with fresh chopped parsley if desired.
- Serve the turmeric roasted sweet potatoes warm as a delicious and flavorful side dish.

Garlic Herb Roasted Asparagus

Ingredients:
- 1 bunch of fresh asparagus
- 2 tablespoons olive oil
- 3 cloves garlic, minced

- 1 teaspoon dried thyme
- 1 teaspoon dried rosemary
- Salt and pepper, to taste
- 1 tablespoon grated Parmesan cheese (optional, for garnish)

Instructions:
- Preheat your oven to 400°F (200°C).
- Wash the asparagus and trim the tough ends. You can do this by holding each end of the asparagus and gently bending it; it will naturally break at the point where it becomes tough. Discard the tough ends.
- In a small bowl, mix together the olive oil, minced garlic, dried thyme, dried rosemary, salt, and pepper.
- Place the trimmed asparagus on a baking sheet lined with parchment paper or aluminum foil.
- Drizzle the garlic and herb mixture over the asparagus, ensuring that each spear is well coated. You can use your hands to toss and evenly coat the asparagus.
- Spread the asparagus in a single layer on the baking sheet for even roasting.
- Roast the asparagus in the preheated oven for about 12-15 minutes, or until the spears are tender but still crisp.
- Optional: Sprinkle grated Parmesan cheese over the roasted asparagus during the last 5 minutes of cooking, allowing it to melt and slightly brown.
- Remove from the oven and serve immediately. You can squeeze a little fresh lemon juice over the asparagus for added brightness if desired.

Sautéed Spinach with Pine Nuts and Raisins

Ingredients:
- 1 pound fresh spinach, washed and trimmed
- 2 tablespoons olive oil
- 2 cloves garlic, minced
- 1/4 cup pine nuts
- 1/4 cup raisins
- Salt and pepper to taste
- Optional: red pepper flakes for some heat
- Lemon wedges for serving

Instructions:
- Rinse the spinach thoroughly and trim any tough stems. If the leaves are large, you can tear them into smaller pieces.

- In a dry skillet over medium heat, toast the pine nuts until they are lightly golden brown. Be careful not to burn them, and stir frequently. Once toasted, remove them from the skillet and set aside.
- In the same skillet, add olive oil and minced garlic. Sauté the garlic over medium heat until it becomes fragrant but not browned.
- Add the prepared spinach to the skillet. Toss and cook until the spinach wilts, which should only take a few minutes. You may need to do this in batches if your skillet is not large enough to accommodate all the spinach at once.
- Once the spinach is wilted, add the toasted pine nuts and raisins to the skillet. Toss everything together until the ingredients are well combined.
- Season the sautéed spinach with salt, pepper, and red pepper flakes if you desire a bit of heat. Adjust the seasoning to your taste.
- Transfer the sautéed spinach to a serving dish. Squeeze some fresh lemon juice over the top before serving.
- Serve the sautéed spinach as a side dish or a light main course. It pairs well with grilled chicken, fish, or as a topping for pasta.

Cucumber Avocado Salad with Lime Dressing

Ingredients:
For the Salad:
- 2 large cucumbers, thinly sliced
- 2 ripe avocados, diced
- 1/2 red onion, thinly sliced
- 1/4 cup fresh cilantro, chopped
- 1/4 cup feta cheese, crumbled (optional)

For the Lime Dressing:
- 3 tablespoons olive oil
- 2 tablespoons fresh lime juice
- 1 teaspoon honey or maple syrup (adjust to taste)
- 1 clove garlic, minced
- Salt and pepper to taste

Instructions:
- Prepare the Vegetables: Slice the cucumbers and red onion thinly. Dice the avocados. If you're using cilantro and feta cheese, chop the cilantro and crumble the feta.
- Combine Ingredients: In a large bowl, combine the sliced cucumbers, diced avocados, sliced red onion, and chopped cilantro. If you're using feta, add it as well.

- Make the Dressing: In a separate small bowl, whisk together the olive oil, lime juice, honey or maple syrup, minced garlic, salt, and pepper. Taste and adjust the sweetness and acidity according to your preference.
- Toss the Salad: Pour the lime dressing over the cucumber, avocado, and other ingredients in the large bowl. Gently toss everything together until the salad is well coated with the dressing.
- Serve: Transfer the salad to a serving platter or individual plates. You can garnish with additional cilantro or feta if desired.
- Enjoy: Serve immediately and enjoy your refreshing Cucumber Avocado Salad with Lime Dressing!

Eggplant Caponata with Olives and Capers

Ingredients:
- 1 large eggplant, diced
- 1 onion, finely chopped
- 2 cloves garlic, minced
- 1 can (14 oz) diced tomatoes
- 1/2 cup green olives, pitted and sliced
- 1/4 cup capers, drained
- 1/4 cup red wine vinegar
- 2 tablespoons tomato paste
- 2 tablespoons sugar
- 1/4 cup fresh basil, chopped
- Salt and pepper, to taste
- Olive oil, for cooking

Instructions:
- Heat a couple of tablespoons of olive oil in a large skillet over medium heat.
- Add the diced eggplant and cook until golden brown and softened. Remove the eggplant from the skillet and set it aside.
- In the same skillet, add a bit more olive oil if needed and sauté the chopped onion until it becomes translucent.
- Add the minced garlic and cook for another minute until fragrant.
- Stir in the diced tomatoes, green olives, and capers. Cook for a few minutes until the tomatoes start to break down.
- In a small bowl, mix together the red wine vinegar, tomato paste, and sugar. Add this mixture to the skillet and stir well.
- Return the cooked eggplant to the skillet and mix everything together. Allow the flavors to meld by cooking for an additional 5-7 minutes.
- Season the caponata with salt and pepper to taste.

- Just before serving, stir in the chopped fresh basil for a burst of flavor.
- Serve the Eggplant Caponata at room temperature or chilled. It's delicious on its own, as a topping for crostini, or as a side dish.

Crispy Baked Kale Chips

Ingredients:
- 1 bunch of kale
- 1-2 tablespoons olive oil
- Salt, to taste
- Optional seasonings: garlic powder, onion powder, paprika, Parmesan cheese, nutritional yeast, etc.

Instructions:
- Preheat your oven to 350°F (175°C).
- Wash the kale thoroughly and dry it completely. Use a salad spinner or pat it dry with a kitchen towel. Remove the tough stems from the kale leaves and tear the leaves into bite-sized pieces.
- Place the torn kale leaves in a large bowl. Drizzle olive oil over the kale, starting with 1 tablespoon. Massage the oil into the kale leaves, ensuring that each leaf is lightly coated. Add more oil if needed, but be careful not to use too much; you want a light coating to avoid sogginess.
- Sprinkle salt over the kale leaves. You can also add optional seasonings like garlic powder, onion powder, paprika, or any other flavors you prefer. Toss the kale again to evenly distribute the seasonings.
- Spread the kale leaves in a single layer on baking sheets. Make sure they are not overcrowded to allow proper crisping.
- Place the baking sheets in the preheated oven. Bake for about 10-15 minutes or until the edges of the kale are crispy and lightly browned. Keep an eye on them, as they can burn quickly.
- Remove the kale chips from the oven and let them cool on the baking sheets for a few minutes. The chips will continue to crisp up as they cool. Once they are cool, transfer them to a serving bowl and enjoy your crispy baked kale chips!

Stuffed Acorn Squash with Quinoa and Cranberries

Ingredients:
- 2 acorn squash, halved and seeds removed
- 1 cup quinoa, rinsed
- 2 cups vegetable broth or water
- 1/2 cup dried cranberries
- 1/2 cup chopped pecans or walnuts

- 1/2 cup chopped fresh parsley
- 1/4 cup olive oil
- 1 onion, finely chopped
- 2 cloves garlic, minced
- 1 teaspoon dried thyme
- Salt and pepper to taste

Instructions:
- Preheat the oven to 375°F (190°C).
- Place the acorn squash halves on a baking sheet, cut side up. Drizzle with olive oil, and season with salt and pepper. Roast in the preheated oven for about 30-40 minutes, or until the squash is fork-tender.
- While the squash is roasting, rinse the quinoa under cold water. In a medium saucepan, combine the quinoa and vegetable broth (or water). Bring to a boil, then reduce the heat to low, cover, and simmer for 15-20 minutes, or until the quinoa is cooked and the liquid is absorbed.
- In a large skillet, heat olive oil over medium heat. Add the chopped onion and garlic, sauté until softened.
- Add the cooked quinoa, dried cranberries, chopped nuts, dried thyme, and chopped parsley to the skillet. Stir to combine, and cook for an additional 5 minutes. Season with salt and pepper, to taste.
- Once the acorn squash is done roasting, stuff each half with the quinoa mixture.
- Return the stuffed squash to the oven and bake for an additional 10-15 minutes, or until the stuffing is heated through and slightly crispy on top.
- Remove from the oven and let it cool for a few minutes before serving.

Steamed Artichokes with Lemon Garlic Aioli

Ingredients:

For Steamed Artichokes:
- 4 large artichokes
- 1 lemon, sliced
- Salt, to taste
- Water for steaming

For Lemon Garlic Aioli:
- 1 cup mayonnaise
- 2 cloves garlic, minced
- 1 tablespoon Dijon mustard
- 1 lemon, juiced
- Salt and pepper, to taste.

Instructions:

For Steamed Artichokes:

Prepare Artichokes:

- Trim the stems of the artichokes and cut off the top 1/4 of each artichoke.
- Use kitchen scissors to trim the sharp tips off the remaining leaves.
- Rub the cut sides of the artichokes with a lemon half to prevent browning.

Steam Artichokes:

- Place a steamer basket in a large pot.
- Fill the pot with water until it's just below the steamer basket.
- Add the sliced lemon to the water.
- Bring the water to a boil.

Steam Artichokes:

- Once boiling, reduce the heat to a simmer.
- Put the prepared artichokes in the steamer basket, cover, and steam for about 25-45 minutes, depending on their size. They are done when a leaf can be easily pulled off.

Serve:

- Let the artichokes cool for a few minutes before serving.
- Serve with lemon garlic aioli for dipping.

For Lemon Garlic Aioli:

- In a small bowl, combine mayonnaise, minced garlic, Dijon mustard, and lemon juice.
- Mix well until all the ingredients are fully incorporated.
- Add salt and pepper to taste.
- Adjust the seasoning if necessary.
- Allow the aioli to chill in the refrigerator for at least 30 minutes before serving to let the flavors meld.
- Serve the lemon garlic aioli alongside the steamed artichokes.

Sesame Ginger Bok Choy

Ingredients:

- 1 pound (about 450g) baby bok choy
- 2 tablespoons sesame oil
- 2 tablespoons soy sauce
- 1 tablespoon rice vinegar
- 1 tablespoon fresh ginger, minced
- 2 cloves garlic, minced
- 1 tablespoon sesame seeds (optional)
- Salt and pepper to taste

Instructions:

Prepare Bok Choy:

- Trim the ends of the baby bok choy and separate the leaves.
- Rinse the leaves thoroughly under cold water to remove any dirt or debris.

Cook Bok Choy:

- Heat sesame oil in a large skillet or wok over medium heat.
- Add minced ginger and garlic to the hot oil and sauté for about 1-2 minutes until fragrant.

Add Bok Choy:

- Add the prepared bok choy leaves to the skillet.
- Stir-fry for 3-5 minutes, tossing the leaves with the ginger and garlic mixture until they begin to wilt.

Season:

- In a small bowl, mix soy sauce and rice vinegar.
- Pour the soy sauce mixture over the bok choy, and toss to coat evenly.
- Season with salt and pepper to taste.

Finish:

- Continue stir-frying for an additional 2-3 minutes or until the bok choy is tender-crisp.
- If desired, sprinkle sesame seeds over the top and toss to combine.

Serve:

- Transfer the sesame ginger bok choy to a serving dish and serve immediately.

Cumin-Roasted Carrot Fries

Ingredients:

- 1 pound (about 450g) carrots, peeled and cut into thin strips or matchsticks
- 2 tablespoons olive oil
- 1 teaspoon ground cumin
- 1/2 teaspoon ground coriander (optional)
- 1/2 teaspoon smoked paprika
- 1/2 teaspoon garlic powder
- 1/2 teaspoon onion powder
- Salt and black pepper to taste
- Fresh parsley or cilantro for garnish (optional)

Instructions:

- Preheat your oven to 425°F (220°C).
- Peel the carrots and cut them into thin strips or matchsticks. Try to make them as uniform as possible for even roasting.
- In a large bowl, combine the olive oil, ground cumin, ground coriander (if using), smoked paprika, garlic powder, onion powder, salt, and black pepper. Mix well to create a uniform seasoning.

- Add the carrot strips to the bowl with the seasoning. Toss the carrots until they are evenly coated with the spice mixture.
- Spread the seasoned carrot strips in a single layer on a baking sheet. Make sure they are not crowded to allow even roasting.
- Place the baking sheet in the preheated oven and roast for about 20-25 minutes or until the carrot fries are golden brown and crispy at the edges. Make sure to toss them halfway through the cooking time for even roasting.
- Once the carrot fries are done, remove them from the oven. If desired, garnish with fresh parsley or cilantro. Serve immediately.
- Consider serving the carrot fries with a dipping sauce of your choice, such as tzatziki, hummus, or a yogurt-based sauce.

Grilled Portobello Mushrooms with Balsamic Glaze

Ingredients:
- 4 large Portobello mushrooms, stems removed
- 2 tablespoons olive oil
- 2 cloves garlic, minced
- Salt and pepper to taste
- 1/4 cup balsamic vinegar
- 2 tablespoons soy sauce (or tamari for a gluten-free option)
- 1 tablespoon honey (or maple syrup for a vegan option)
- Fresh parsley, chopped, for garnish (optional)

Instructions:
- Preheat the grill to medium-high heat.
- Clean the Portobello mushrooms with a damp cloth or paper towel. Remove the stems and set aside.
- In a small bowl, whisk together the olive oil, minced garlic, salt, and pepper. Brush the mushroom caps on both sides with the mixture.
- In another bowl, combine balsamic vinegar, soy sauce, and honey. Mix well to create the glaze.
- Place the mushrooms on the preheated grill, cap side down. Grill for about 5-7 minutes per side, or until the mushrooms are tender and have grill marks.
- During the last 2-3 minutes of grilling, brush the tops of the mushrooms with the balsamic glaze.
- Once the mushrooms are cooked through and have absorbed the flavors, remove them from the grill.
- Drizzle the remaining balsamic glaze over the grilled mushrooms and garnish with chopped fresh parsley if desired.

- Serve the grilled Portobello mushrooms immediately as a delicious side dish or as a main course. They can be enjoyed on their own or as a topping for salads, burgers, or sandwiches.

Herbed Cauliflower Rice

Ingredients:
- 1 head of cauliflower
- 2 tablespoons olive oil
- 2 cloves garlic, minced
- 1 teaspoon dried thyme
- 1 teaspoon dried rosemary
- 1/2 teaspoon dried oregano
- Salt and pepper to taste
- Fresh parsley, chopped (for garnish, optional)

Instructions:
Prepare the Cauliflower:
- Remove the leaves and stem from the cauliflower, and cut it into florets.
- Use a food processor to pulse the cauliflower until it resembles the texture of rice. You can also use a box grater if you don't have a food processor.

Cook the Cauliflower Rice:
- In a large skillet or pan, heat the olive oil over medium heat.
- Add the minced garlic and sauté for about 1 minute until it becomes fragrant.

Add Cauliflower Rice:
- Add the riced cauliflower to the skillet. Stir well to coat the cauliflower with the garlic and olive oil.

Season with Herbs:
- Sprinkle the dried thyme, rosemary, and oregano over the cauliflower rice.
- Season with salt and pepper to taste. Stir to combine.

Cooking Process:
- Cook the cauliflower rice for about 5-7 minutes, stirring occasionally. The goal is to cook it until it's tender but not mushy.

Serve:
- Once the cauliflower rice is cooked, remove it from heat.
- Garnish with fresh chopped parsley if desired.

Enjoy:
- Serve the herbed cauliflower rice as a side dish with your favorite protein or use it as a base for other dishes.

Broccoli and Cheddar Stuffed Spaghetti Squash

Ingredients:

- 1 medium-sized spaghetti squash
- 2 cups broccoli florets, steamed
- 1 cup shredded cheddar cheese
- 2 tablespoons olive oil
- 2 cloves garlic, minced
- Salt and pepper to taste
- 1 teaspoon dried oregano
- 1 teaspoon dried basil
- Optional: Red pepper flakes for some heat
- Fresh parsley for garnish (optional)

Instructions:

- Preheat your oven to 400°F (200°C).
- Cut the spaghetti squash in half lengthwise. Scoop out the seeds and pulp from the center using a spoon.
- Brush the cut sides of the squash with olive oil and season with salt and pepper.
- Place the squash halves, cut side down, on a baking sheet lined with parchment paper. Bake in the preheated oven for about 40-45 minutes, or until the squash is tender and easily pierced with a fork.
- While the squash is baking, heat 2 tablespoons of olive oil in a skillet over medium heat. Add minced garlic and sauté until fragrant.
- Add steamed broccoli florets to the skillet and toss to combine with the garlic. Season with salt, pepper, dried oregano, and dried basil. Cook for 2-3 minutes until the broccoli is heated through.
- Once the spaghetti squash is done baking, use a fork to scrape the inside of each half, creating "spaghetti" strands. Leave the squash strands inside the shells.
- Mix the spaghetti squash strands with the broccoli mixture in the skillet.
- Divide the mixture evenly between the squash halves, pressing it down slightly.
- Sprinkle shredded cheddar cheese over the top of each stuffed squash half.
- Place the stuffed squash back in the oven and bake for an additional 10-15 minutes, or until the cheese is melted and bubbly.
- Optional: Garnish with red pepper flakes and fresh parsley before serving.

Diabetes-Friendly Desserts Recipes

Avocado Chocolate Mousse

Ingredients:
- 2 ripe avocados
- 1/3 cup cocoa powder (unsweetened)
- 1/3 cup maple syrup or honey (adjust to taste)
- 1/3 cup milk (dairy or plant-based)
- 1 teaspoon vanilla extract
- A pinch of salt
- Optional toppings: whipped cream, berries, or shaved chocolate

Instructions:
- Cut the avocados in half and remove the pits.
- Scoop the flesh into a blender or food processor.
- Add cocoa powder, maple syrup or honey, milk, vanilla extract, and a pinch of salt to the blender or food processor with the avocados.
- Blend until the mixture is smooth and creamy. You may need to stop and scrape down the sides to ensure everything is well combined.
- Taste the mousse and adjust the sweetness if necessary by adding more maple syrup or honey. Blend again to combine.
- If you prefer a chilled mousse, refrigerate the mixture for at least 1-2 hours before serving.
- Spoon the avocado chocolate mousse into serving glasses or bowls.
- Garnish with whipped cream, berries, or shaved chocolate, if desired.
- Serve and enjoy your delicious and healthy avocado chocolate mousse!

Almond Flour Blueberry Muffins

Ingredients:
- 2 cups almond flour
- 1/4 cup coconut flour
- 1/2 teaspoon baking soda
- 1/4 teaspoon salt
- 3 large eggs
- 1/3 cup honey or maple syrup
- 1/4 cup melted coconut oil or melted butter
- 1 teaspoon vanilla extract
- 1 cup fresh or frozen blueberries

Instructions:

- Preheat your oven to 350°F (175°C). Line a muffin tin with paper liners or grease it well.
- In a large bowl, whisk together the almond flour, coconut flour, baking soda, and salt.
- In another bowl, beat the eggs. Add honey (or maple syrup), melted coconut oil (or melted butter), and vanilla extract. Mix well.
- Add the wet ingredients to the dry ingredients and stir until well combined.
- Gently fold in the blueberries. If you're using frozen blueberries, you can toss them in a bit of almond flour before adding them to the batter to prevent them from sinking to the bottom.
- Spoon the batter into the prepared muffin tin, filling each cup about 2/3 full.
- Bake in the preheated oven for 18-22 minutes, or until a toothpick inserted into the center of a muffin comes out clean.
- Allow the muffins to cool in the tin for 5 minutes, then transfer them to a wire rack to cool completely.

Cinnamon Baked Pears

Ingredients:

- 4 ripe but firm pears
- 2 tablespoons unsalted butter, melted
- 3 tablespoons brown sugar
- 1 teaspoon ground cinnamon
- 1/4 teaspoon ground nutmeg
- 1/4 teaspoon vanilla extract
- 1/4 cup chopped nuts (such as walnuts or pecans), optional
- Vanilla ice cream or whipped cream for serving, optional

Instructions:

- Preheat your oven to 375°F (190°C).
- Wash and peel the pears. Cut them in half lengthwise and remove the cores using a melon baller or spoon, creating a hollow indentation.
- In a small bowl, mix together the melted butter, brown sugar, cinnamon, nutmeg, and vanilla extract.
- Place the pear halves in a baking dish, cut side up. Brush or drizzle the melted butter and sugar mixture over the pears, making sure to coat them evenly.
- If using nuts, sprinkle them over the top of the pears.
- Bake the pears in the preheated oven for about 25-30 minutes, or until the pears are tender and the tops are golden brown.
- Remove the baked pears from the oven and let them cool slightly before serving. You can serve them as is or with a scoop of vanilla ice cream or a dollop of whipped cream for an extra treat.

- Enjoy your delicious cinnamon baked pears!

Chia Seed Pudding Parfait

Ingredients:
- For Chia Seed Pudding:
- 1/4 cup chia seeds
- 1 cup almond milk (or any milk of your choice)
- 1-2 tablespoons maple syrup or honey (adjust to taste)
- 1/2 teaspoon vanilla extract

For Parfait Layers:
- 1 cup Greek yogurt (or plant-based yogurt for a vegan option)
- Fresh fruits (berries, kiwi, banana slices, etc.)
- Granola
- Nuts (sliced almonds, chopped walnuts, etc.)

Instructions:

Prepare Chia Seed Pudding:
- In a bowl, mix chia seeds, almond milk, maple syrup (or honey), and vanilla extract.
- Stir well to ensure the chia seeds are evenly distributed.
- Cover the bowl and refrigerate for at least 4 hours or overnight, allowing the chia seeds to absorb the liquid and create a pudding-like consistency.

Assemble the Parfait:
- Take serving glasses or jars.
- Start by layering the bottom with a spoonful of chia seed pudding.

Add Yogurt Layer:
- Add a layer of Greek yogurt on top of the chia seed pudding.

Fruit Layer:
- Add a layer of fresh fruit. You can use a variety of berries, sliced kiwi, or banana slices.

Granola Layer:
- Sprinkle a layer of granola over the fruits.

Repeat Layers:
- Repeat the layers until you reach the top of the glass or jar. You can customize the layers according to your preferences.

Top with Nuts:
- Finish the parfait by topping it with a sprinkle of sliced almonds, chopped walnuts, or your favorite nuts.

Serve:
- Serve the Chia Seed Pudding Parfait immediately, and enjoy the delightful combination of textures and flavors!

Sugar-Free Apple Crisp

Ingredients:
For the Filling:
- 6 cups peeled, cored, and sliced apples (such as Granny Smith or Honeycrisp)
- 1 tablespoon lemon juice
- 1 teaspoon ground cinnamon
- 1/4 teaspoon nutmeg
- 1/4 cup unsweetened applesauce
- 2 tablespoons cornstarch or arrowroot powder

For the Topping:
- 1 cup old-fashioned rolled oats
- 1/2 cup almond flour
- 1/4 cup chopped nuts (such as walnuts or pecans)
- 1 teaspoon ground cinnamon
- 1/4 cup melted coconut oil or unsweetened applesauce
- 1/4 teaspoon salt

Instructions:
- Preheat your oven to 350°F (175°C).
- In a large mixing bowl, combine the sliced apples with lemon juice, cinnamon, nutmeg, applesauce, and cornstarch. Toss until the apples are evenly coated.
- Transfer the apple mixture to a greased baking dish and spread it out evenly.
- In a separate bowl, combine the oats, almond flour, chopped nuts, cinnamon, melted coconut oil or applesauce, and salt. Mix until the topping is well combined.
- Sprinkle the topping evenly over the apple mixture in the baking dish.
- Bake in the preheated oven for 35-40 minutes, or until the topping is golden brown and the apples are tender.
- Remove it from the oven and let it cool for a few minutes before serving.
- Optionally, serve with a dollop of sugar-free whipped cream or a scoop of sugar-free vanilla ice cream.

Coconut Flour Lemon Bars

Ingredients:
For the Crust:
- 1 cup coconut flour
- 1/2 cup melted coconut oil
- 1/4 cup honey or maple syrup
- 1/2 teaspoon vanilla extract
- A pinch of salt

For the Lemon Filling:
- 4 large eggs
- 1 cup fresh lemon juice (about 4-5 lemons)
- 1/2 cup honey or maple syrup
- 1/4 cup coconut flour
- Zest of 1 lemon

Instructions:

Preheat the Oven:
- Preheat your oven to 350°F (175°C). Grease a square baking dish (8x8 inches or similar size) and line it with parchment paper, leaving some overhang for easy removal.

Make the Crust:
- In a mixing bowl, combine the coconut flour, melted coconut oil, honey or maple syrup, vanilla extract, and a pinch of salt.
- Mix until well combined, and press the mixture evenly into the bottom of the prepared baking dish.
- Bake the crust in the preheated oven for about 10-12 minutes, or until it's just beginning to turn golden around the edges.

Prepare the Lemon Filling:
- In a separate bowl, whisk together the eggs, fresh lemon juice, honey or maple syrup, coconut flour, and lemon zest until smooth.
- Pour the lemon filling over the pre-baked crust.

Bake the Bars:
- Return the baking dish to the oven and bake for an additional 20-25 minutes, or until the filling is set and the edges are golden.
- Remove from the oven and let it cool in the dish for about 30 minutes.

Chill and Serve:
- Once cooled, transfer the lemon bars to the refrigerator and let them chill for at least 2 hours or until fully set.
- Once set, use the parchment paper overhang to lift the bars out of the dish and onto a cutting board.
- Cut into squares or bars, and serve. Optionally, dust with coconut flour or powdered sugar for decoration.

Pumpkin Spice Energy Bites

Ingredients:
- 1 cup old-fashioned oats
- 1/2 cup pumpkin puree
- 1/4 cup honey or maple syrup
- 1/2 cup almond butter (or any nut butter of your choice)

- 1/3 cup shredded coconut (unsweetened)
- 1/2 teaspoon vanilla extract
- 1 teaspoon pumpkin spice mix (cinnamon, nutmeg, ginger, and cloves)
- A pinch of salt
- Optional: 1/4 cup mini chocolate chips or chopped nuts for added texture

Instructions:
- In a large mixing bowl, combine the oats, pumpkin puree, honey (or maple syrup), almond butter, shredded coconut, vanilla extract, pumpkin spice mix, and a pinch of salt.
- Mix the ingredients well until everything is evenly combined. If the mixture seems too wet, you can add a bit more oats. If it's too dry, you can add a little more pumpkin puree or nut butter.
- If you choose to add chocolate chips or nuts, fold them into the mixture.
- Once the mixture is well combined, refrigerate it for about 30 minutes. Chilling the mixture makes it easier to handle.
- After chilling, take small portions of the mixture and roll them into bite-sized balls using your hands.
- Place the energy bites on a parchment-lined tray and refrigerate for at least another 30 minutes to firm up.
- Once the energy bites are firm, transfer them to an airtight container and store them in the refrigerator. They can be enjoyed for up to a week.

Walnut and Cinnamon Baked Apples

Ingredients:
- 4 medium-sized apples (such as Granny Smith or Honeycrisp)
- 1/2 cup chopped walnuts
- 1/4 cup brown sugar
- 1 teaspoon ground cinnamon
- 1/4 teaspoon nutmeg
- 2 tablespoons unsalted butter, melted
- 1/2 cup apple juice or water

Instructions:
- Preheat your oven to 375°F (190°C).
- Wash and core the apples, leaving the bottoms intact so the filling stays inside.
- In a bowl, mix together the chopped walnuts, brown sugar, ground cinnamon, and nutmeg.
- Stuff each cored apple with the walnut mixture, pressing down gently.
- Place the stuffed apples in a baking dish. Drizzle the melted butter over the top of each apple.

- Pour apple juice or water into the bottom of the baking dish to prevent the apples from drying out during baking.
- Bake the apples in the preheated oven for about 30-40 minutes or until they are tender. The baking time may vary depending on the size and type of apples, so check for doneness by inserting a fork into the apples.
- Once baked, remove the apples from the oven and let them cool for a few minutes. You can serve them warm as they are or with a scoop of vanilla ice cream for an extra treat.

Keto Chocolate Avocado Pudding

Ingredients:
- 2 ripe avocados
- 1/4 cup unsweetened cocoa powder
- 1/4 cup almond milk (unsweetened)
- 1/4 cup heavy cream
- 1/4 cup powdered erythritol (adjust to taste)
- 1 teaspoon vanilla extract
- A pinch of salt

Instructions:
- Cut the avocados in half, remove the pits, and scoop the flesh into a blender or food processor.
- Blend the avocados until smooth and creamy.
- Add the unsweetened cocoa powder to the blender.
- Pour in the almond milk and heavy cream.
- Add the powdered erythritol to the mixture. Adjust the amount based on your sweetness preference.
- Add the vanilla extract to enhance the flavor.
- Add a pinch of salt to balance the flavors.
- Blend all the ingredients until well combined and the mixture is smooth.
- Taste the pudding and adjust the sweetness or cocoa powder if needed.
- Transfer the pudding to a bowl or individual serving cups and refrigerate for at least 1-2 hours to allow it to firm up.
- Once chilled, you can serve the keto chocolate avocado pudding as is or garnish with whipped cream, nuts, or berries if desired.

Berry and Almond Yogurt Parfait

Ingredients:
- 1 cup Greek yogurt
- 1 cup mixed berries (strawberries, blueberries, raspberries, etc.)
- 1/2 cup granola

- 1/4 cup sliced almonds
- 2 tablespoons honey or maple syrup (optional, for sweetness)
- Fresh mint leaves for garnish (optional)

Instructions:
- In a bowl, mix the Greek yogurt with honey or maple syrup if you want it sweeter. Adjust sweetness to your liking.
- Start by placing a spoonful of the sweetened yogurt at the bottom of your serving glasses or bowls.
- Add a layer of mixed berries on top of the yogurt. You can either mix the berries or layer them individually.
- Sprinkle a layer of granola over the berries. This adds a crunchy texture to the parfait.
- Repeat the process by adding another layer of yogurt, followed by berries, and then granola until you reach the top of the glass or bowl.
- Finish the parfait by sprinkling sliced almonds on top. This adds a nutty flavor and crunch.
- Optionally, garnish the parfait with fresh mint leaves for a burst of freshness.
- Serve immediately and enjoy your delicious Berry and Almond Yogurt Parfait!

Vanilla Chia Seed Coconut Pudding

Ingredients:
- 1/4 cup chia seeds
- 1 cup coconut milk (you can use canned or homemade)
- 1 teaspoon pure vanilla extract
- 1-2 tablespoons maple syrup or honey (adjust to taste)
- Optional toppings: sliced fruits, shredded coconut, nuts

Instructions:
- In a bowl, combine the chia seeds, coconut milk, vanilla extract, and sweetener. Whisk well to ensure that the chia seeds are evenly distributed.
- Let the mixture sit for about 5 minutes, and then whisk again to prevent clumps. This initial waiting period allows the chia seeds to absorb some liquid.
- Cover the bowl and refrigerate the mixture for at least 2-3 hours, or preferably overnight. During this time, the chia seeds will absorb the liquid and form a pudding-like consistency.
- Before serving, give the pudding a good stir. If it's too thick, you can add a little more coconut milk to reach your desired consistency.
- Taste the pudding and adjust the sweetness if needed by adding more maple syrup or honey.

- Serve the vanilla chia seed coconut pudding in individual bowls or jars. Top with sliced fruits, shredded coconut, or nuts for added flavor and texture.
- Enjoy your delicious and nutritious Vanilla Chia Seed Coconut Pudding!

Sugar-Free Cheesecake Bites

Ingredients:

For the Crust:
- 1 cup almond flour
- 3 tablespoons melted butter (unsalted)
- 1 tablespoon granulated sugar substitute (like erythritol or stevia)

For the Cheesecake Filling:
- 8 ounces cream cheese, softened
- 1/2 cup sour cream
- 1/3 cup granulated sugar substitute
- 1 teaspoon vanilla extract
- 2 large eggs

Instructions:

Crust:
- Preheat your oven to 325°F (163°C). Line a mini muffin tin with paper liners.
- In a medium bowl, combine almond flour, melted butter, and sugar substitute for the crust. Mix until well combined.
- Press about 1 tablespoon of the crust mixture into the bottom of each mini muffin cup. Use the back of a spoon to compact the crust.
- Bake the crusts in the preheated oven for 8-10 minutes, or until they are just starting to turn golden.
- Remove them from the oven and let them cool while you prepare the cheesecake filling.

Cheesecake Filling:
- In a large mixing bowl, beat the softened cream cheese until smooth and creamy.
- Add the sour cream, sugar substitute, and vanilla extract to the cream cheese. Mix until well combined and smooth.
- Add the eggs one at a time, beating well after each addition. Continue to beat until the mixture is smooth and creamy.
- Spoon or pipe the cheesecake filling over the cooled crusts in the mini muffin tin.
- Bake in the preheated oven for 12-15 minutes, or until the cheesecake is set and the edges are just starting to turn golden.
- Allow the cheesecake bites to cool in the muffin tin, then transfer them to the refrigerator to chill for at least 2 hours before serving.

- Once chilled, remove the cheesecake bites from the muffin tin and enjoy your delicious sugar-free cheesecake bites!

Raspberry Almond Thumbprint Cookies

Ingredients:
- 1 cup (2 sticks) unsalted butter, softened
- 2/3 cup granulated sugar
- 1/2 teaspoon almond extract
- 2 cups all-purpose flour
- 1/2 cup finely ground almonds
- 1/2 teaspoon salt
- 1/2 cup raspberry jam or preserves
- Sliced almonds for garnish (optional)
- Powdered sugar for dusting (optional)

Instructions:
- Preheat your oven to 350°F (175°C). Line baking sheets with parchment paper.
- In a large mixing bowl, cream together the softened butter and granulated sugar until light and fluffy.
- Add the almond extract to the butter and sugar mixture and mix well.
- In a separate bowl, whisk together the flour, ground almonds, and salt.
- Gradually add the dry ingredients to the butter mixture, mixing until just combined. Be careful not to overmix.
- Shape the dough into 1-inch balls and place them on the prepared baking sheets, spacing them about 2 inches apart.
- Use your thumb or the back of a spoon to make an indentation in the center of each cookie.
- Fill each indentation with a small amount of raspberry jam or preserve. Don't overfill to avoid the jam overflowing during baking.
- Optional: Place a sliced almond on top of each cookie for garnish.
- Bake in the preheated oven for 12-15 minutes, or until the edges are lightly golden.
- Allow the cookies to cool on the baking sheets for a few minutes before transferring them to a wire rack to cool completely.
- Optional: Dust the cooled cookies with powdered sugar for a decorative touch.

Cocoa-Dusted Almonds

Ingredients:
- 2 cups whole almonds
- 1/4 cup cocoa powder
- 1/4 cup powdered sugar

- 1/2 teaspoon vanilla extract
- 1/4 teaspoon salt
- 1 tablespoon water

Instructions:

Roast the Almonds:
- Preheat your oven to 350°F (175°C).
- Spread the almonds evenly on a baking sheet.
- Roast the almonds in the preheated oven for about 10-15 minutes, or until they become fragrant and slightly golden. Stir them occasionally for even roasting.

Prepare the Cocoa Coating:
- In a small bowl, whisk together the cocoa powder, powdered sugar, vanilla extract, salt, and water.
- Mix until you have a smooth, thick paste.

Coat the Almonds:
- Once the almonds are roasted and still warm, transfer them to a large mixing bowl.
- Pour the cocoa mixture over the warm almonds and toss them until all the almonds are evenly coated.

Cooling and Separating:
- Spread the cocoa-dusted almonds back onto the baking sheet in a single layer.
- Allow them to cool completely, and the coating will harden as it cools.

Serve or Store:
- Once the almonds are completely cooled and the coating is set, they are ready to be served.
- Store in an airtight container at room temperature for up to two weeks.

Lemon Coconut Bliss Balls

Ingredients:
- 1 cup shredded coconut (plus extra for coating)
- 1 cup raw cashews
- 1 cup pitted dates
- Zest of 1 lemon
- 2 tablespoons fresh lemon juice
- 1 tablespoon coconut oil (melted)
- 1 teaspoon vanilla extract
- A pinch of salt

Instructions:
- If the dates are not soft, soak them in warm water for about 10 minutes and then drain.

- Zest the lemon and squeeze the juice.
- In a food processor, blend the raw cashews until they form a fine crumb.
- Add the pitted dates, shredded coconut, lemon zest, lemon juice, melted coconut oil, vanilla extract, and a pinch of salt to the food processor with the cashews.
- Blend the ingredients until they come together into a sticky, dough-like consistency. You should be able to pinch the mixture, and it should hold together.
- Take small portions of the mixture and roll them between your palms to form small bliss balls. You can make them any size you prefer.
- Roll the bliss balls in shredded coconut to coat them evenly.
- Place the bliss balls in the refrigerator for at least 30 minutes to firm up.
- Once chilled, your Lemon Coconut Bliss Balls are ready to be enjoyed! They make a delicious and healthy snack.
- Store the bliss balls in an airtight container in the refrigerator for up to two weeks. You can also freeze them for longer storage.

Sugar-Free Pistachio Ice Cream

This recipe uses an ice cream maker, but if you don't have one, you can still make it by placing the mixture in a shallow dish in the freezer and stirring every 30 minutes until it reaches the desired consistency.

Ingredients:
- 2 cups unsalted, shelled pistachios
- 2 cups unsweetened almond milk (or any other unsweetened milk of your choice)
- 1 cup heavy cream
- 1/2 cup powdered erythritol or another sugar substitute (adjust to taste)
- 1 teaspoon vanilla extract
- A pinch of salt

Instructions:
Prepare the Pistachios:
- Preheat your oven to 350°F (175°C).
- Spread the pistachios on a baking sheet and roast them in the oven for about 8-10 minutes, or until they are fragrant. Be careful not to burn them.
- Allow the pistachios to cool, then roughly chop or process them in a food processor until you achieve a coarse texture.

Make the Pistachio Paste:
- Set aside about 1/2 cup of chopped pistachios for later.
- Take the remaining pistachios and blend them in a food processor until you get a smooth paste. This may take a few minutes, and you may need to scrape down the sides of the processor occasionally.

Prepare the Ice Cream Base:

- In a mixing bowl, combine the pistachio paste, almond milk, heavy cream, powdered erythritol (or your chosen sugar substitute), vanilla extract, and a pinch of salt.
- Mix well until everything is thoroughly combined.

Chill the Mixture:

- Cover the bowl and refrigerate the mixture for at least 2-4 hours, or overnight. This allows the flavors to meld and the mixture to cool, making it easier to churn.

Churn the Ice Cream:

- Transfer the chilled mixture to your ice cream maker and churn according to the manufacturer's instructions. This typically takes about 20-30 minutes.

Add Chopped Pistachios:

- During the last few minutes of churning, add the reserved chopped pistachios to the ice cream maker. This will distribute the nutty texture throughout the ice cream.

Transfer and Freeze:

- Transfer the churned ice cream to a lidded container, smoothing the top with a spatula.
- Freeze the ice cream for at least 4-6 hours or until it reaches your desired firmness.

Now you have delicious sugar-free pistachio ice cream ready to enjoy! Feel free to adjust the sweetness to your liking by adding more or less of the sugar substitute.

Spiced Pumpkin Seeds

Ingredients:

- 2 cups raw pumpkin seeds (also known as pepitas)
- 1 tablespoon olive oil
- 1 teaspoon ground cumin
- 1 teaspoon paprika
- 1/2 teaspoon cayenne pepper (adjust to taste)
- 1/2 teaspoon garlic powder
- 1/2 teaspoon onion powder
- 1/2 teaspoon salt (adjust to taste)
- 1/4 teaspoon black pepper

Instructions:

- Preheat your oven to 300°F (150°C).
- Rinse the pumpkin seeds under cold water to remove any pulp. Pat them dry with a paper towel.
- In a bowl, mix together the olive oil, ground cumin, paprika, cayenne pepper, garlic powder, onion powder, salt, and black pepper. Adjust the seasonings according to your taste preferences.
- Toss the dry pumpkin seeds in the seasoning mixture, ensuring they are well-coated.

- Spread the seasoned pumpkin seeds in a single layer on a baking sheet. Make sure they are evenly distributed.
- Bake the pumpkin seeds in the preheated oven for about 20-25 minutes or until they are golden brown and crispy. Stir the seeds halfway through the baking time to ensure even roasting.
- Allow the spiced pumpkin seeds to cool on the baking sheet for a few minutes. They will continue to crisp up as they cool.
- Once the pumpkin seeds are completely cool, transfer them to an airtight container. Enjoy these spiced pumpkin seeds as a snack or use them as a topping for salads or soups.

Chocolate Avocado Truffles

Ingredients:
- 1 ripe avocado
- 1 cup dark chocolate chips or chopped dark chocolate (70% cocoa or higher)
- 2-3 tablespoons cocoa powder (for coating)
- 2 tablespoons maple syrup or honey (adjust to taste)
- 1 teaspoon vanilla extract
- A pinch of salt

Instructions:
- In a heatproof bowl, melt the dark chocolate either using a double boiler or by microwaving it in 30-second intervals, stirring each time until smooth. Be careful not to overheat.
- Cut the ripe avocado in half, remove the pit, and scoop out the flesh. Mash the avocado in a bowl until smooth.
- Add the melted chocolate, maple syrup (or honey), vanilla extract, and a pinch of salt to the mashed avocado. Mix well until all the ingredients are thoroughly combined.
- Place the mixture in the refrigerator for at least 30 minutes or until it becomes firm enough to handle.
- Once the mixture is firm, use a spoon to scoop out small portions and roll them into bite-sized truffle balls. Place them on a parchment paper-lined tray.
- Roll each truffle in cocoa powder to coat them evenly. This adds a nice finish and prevents them from sticking.
- If the truffles have become too soft during the rolling process, you can chill them again for a short time before serving.
- Your Chocolate Avocado Truffles are now ready to be enjoyed! Store them in the refrigerator until serving.

Raspberry Chia Seed Jam

Ingredients:
- 3 cups fresh or frozen raspberries
- 1/4 cup maple syrup or honey (adjust to taste)
- 2-3 tablespoons chia seeds (add more for thicker jam)
- 1 teaspoon vanilla extract (optional)

Instructions:
- If using fresh raspberries, wash them thoroughly. If using frozen raspberries, allow them to thaw slightly.
- In a medium-sized saucepan, add the raspberries and cook over medium heat. Use a fork or potato masher to crush the berries as they cook.
- Add the maple syrup or honey to the crushed raspberries. Stir well to combine. Taste and adjust the sweetness according to your preference.
- Bring the raspberry mixture to a gentle simmer over medium heat. Allow it to cook for about 5-10 minutes, stirring occasionally. The raspberries should break down and the mixture will thicken.
- Reduce the heat to low, and stir in the chia seeds. Continue to cook and stir for another 5 minutes. The chia seeds will absorb the liquid and help thicken the jam.
- If desired, add vanilla extract to enhance the flavor. Stir well.
- Remove the saucepan from heat and let the jam cool to room temperature. As it cools, it will thicken further.
- Once the jam has cooled, transfer it to sterilized glass jars or containers. Seal the jars and refrigerate.
- Enjoy your homemade raspberry chia seed jam on toast, yogurt, pancakes, or as a topping for desserts.

Diabetes-Friendly Smoothie Recipes

Berry Blast Smoothie

Ingredients:

- 1/2 cup blueberries
- 1/2 cup strawberries, hulled and sliced
- 1/4 cup raspberries
- 1 cup unsweetened almond milk
- Ice cubes

Instructions:

- Wash the blueberries, strawberries, and raspberries thoroughly.
- Hull and slice the strawberries.
- In a blender, combine the blueberries, sliced strawberries, raspberries, and unsweetened almond milk.
- Add a handful of ice cubes to the blender for a refreshing chill.
- Blend the ingredients on high speed until smooth and well combined.
- If the smoothie is too thick, you can add more almond milk to achieve your desired consistency.
- Taste the smoothie and adjust sweetness if necessary. If you prefer a sweeter smoothie, you can add a sweetener of your choice, such as honey or agave syrup.
- Once the desired consistency and taste are achieved, pour the Berry Blast Smoothie into glasses and serve immediately.
- Optionally, garnish with a few whole berries on top for a decorative touch.

Green Power Smoothie

Ingredients:

- 1 cup spinach leaves
- 1/2 cucumber, peeled and sliced
- 1/2 green apple, cored
- 1 tablespoon chia seeds
- 1 cup water

Instructions:

- Prepare the Ingredients: Wash the spinach leaves thoroughly. Peel and slice the cucumber. Core and chop the green apple.
- Assemble in Blender: Place the spinach leaves, sliced cucumber, chopped green apple, and chia seeds in a blender.
- Add Water: Pour 1 cup of water into the blender.

- Blend Until Smooth: Secure the blender lid and blend the ingredients until you achieve a smooth consistency. This might take a minute or two, depending on the power of your blender.
- Check Consistency: If the smoothie is too thick, you can add more water in small increments and blend again until you reach your desired consistency.
- Serve Immediately: Pour the green power smoothie into a glass and enjoy it immediately to benefit from its freshness and nutritional value.

Avocado Delight Smoothie

Ingredients:
- 1/2 ripe avocado
- 1/2 cup spinach
- 1/2 cup cucumber
- 1 tablespoon flaxseeds
- 1 cup water or unsweetened almond milk

Instructions:
- Peel and pit the ripe avocado.
- Wash the spinach and cucumber.
- In a blender, combine the ripe avocado, spinach, cucumber, and flaxseeds.
- Add 1 cup of water or unsweetened almond milk to the blender.
- Blend the ingredients until smooth and creamy.
- If the smoothie is too thick, you can add more water or almond milk in small increments until you reach your desired consistency.
- Pour the smoothie into a glass, sit back, and enjoy!

Tropical Paradise Smoothie:

Ingredients:
- 1/2 cup pineapple chunks
- 1/2 cup mango chunks
- 1/2 banana
- 1 cup coconut water
- Ice cubes

Instructions:
- Peel and chop the pineapple into chunks.
- Peel and chop the mango into chunks.
- Peel and slice the banana.
- Place the pineapple chunks, mango chunks, banana slices, and ice cubes into a blender.
- Pour 1 cup of coconut water into the blender.

- Secure the blender lid tightly.
- Start blending on low speed and gradually increase to high.
- Blend until the mixture is smooth and has a creamy consistency.
- If the smoothie is too thick, you can add more coconut water and blend again until you reach the desired consistency.
- Pour the smoothie into glasses.
- Garnish with a slice of pineapple or a wedge of mango on the rim of the glass for a decorative touch. (Optional)
- Serve immediately and enjoy your refreshing Tropical Paradise Smoothie!

Cinnamon Apple Pie Smoothie

Ingredients:
- 1/2 cup chopped apple (with skin)
- 1/2 teaspoon cinnamon
- 1/4 teaspoon nutmeg
- 1 cup unsweetened soy milk
- Ice cubes

Instructions:
- Begin by gathering all the ingredients.
- In a blender, combine the chopped apple, cinnamon, nutmeg, and unsweetened soy milk.
- Add a handful of ice cubes to the blender. The amount of ice cubes can be adjusted based on personal preference for thickness and coldness.
- Blend the mixture until it reaches a smooth consistency. This may take a minute or two, depending on the power of your blender.
- Once the smoothie is well-blended, pour it into a glass.
- Optionally, you can garnish the smoothie with a sprinkle of cinnamon on top or a slice of apple for presentation.
- Enjoy your delicious and nutritious Cinnamon Apple Pie Smoothie!

Berries and Greek Yogurt Smoothie

Ingredients:
- 1/2 cup mixed berries (blueberries, strawberries)
- 1/2 cup Greek yogurt (unsweetened)
- 1 tablespoon chia seeds
- 1 cup water

Instructions:
- Gather the ingredients: mixed berries, Greek yogurt, chia seeds, and water.

- Measure 1/2 cup of mixed berries (you can use a combination of blueberries and strawberries).
- Measure 1/2 cup of unsweetened Greek yogurt.
- Add 1 tablespoon of chia seeds to the mix.
- Pour 1 cup of water into the blender.
- Blend the ingredients until well combined. This usually takes a minute or two, depending on the power of your blender.
- Once the smoothie reaches a smooth and creamy consistency, stop the blender.
- Pour the smoothie into a glass and enjoy your refreshing and nutritious berries and Greek yogurt smoothie!

Cherry Almond Smoothie

Ingredients:
- 1/2 cup pitted cherries
- 1 tablespoon almond butter
- 1/2 cup spinach leaves
- 1 cup unsweetened almond milk
- Ice cubes

Instructions:
- Make sure the cherries are pitted.
- In a blender, combine the pitted cherries, almond butter, spinach leaves, and unsweetened almond milk.
- Add a handful of ice cubes to the blender.
- Blend the ingredients until smooth and creamy.
- Pour the cherry almond smoothie into a glass and enjoy immediately.

Peanut Butter Banana Bliss

Ingredients:
- 1/2 banana
- 1 tablespoon natural peanut butter
- 1/2 cup spinach leaves
- 1 cup water or unsweetened soy milk

Instructions:
- Peel and slice the banana into smaller pieces for easier blending.
- Measure 1 tablespoon of natural peanut butter.
- Measure 1/2 cup of fresh spinach leaves.
- Place the banana slices, natural peanut butter, and spinach leaves in a blender.

- Pour 1 cup of water or unsweetened soy milk into the blender. Adjust the quantity based on your desired consistency; more liquid for a thinner smoothie, less for a thicker one.
- Secure the lid on the blender and blend the ingredients until smooth. This usually takes about 30 seconds to 1 minute, depending on the power of your blender.
- After blending, check the consistency of the smoothie. If it's too thick, you can add more liquid and blend again until you reach your desired texture.
- Pour the Peanut Butter Banana Bliss into a glass and enjoy immediately!

Carrot Cake Smoothie

Ingredients:
- 1/2 cup shredded carrots
- 1/2 apple, cored
- 1/4 teaspoon cinnamon
- 1/4 teaspoon nutmeg
- 1 cup water or unsweetened almond milk
- Ice cubes

Instructions:
- Peel and shred 1/2 cup of carrots.
- Core and chop 1/2 of an apple.
- Place the shredded carrots and chopped apple into a blender.
- Add 1/4 teaspoon of cinnamon to the blender.
- Add 1/4 teaspoon of nutmeg to the blender.
- Pour 1 cup of water or unsweetened almond milk into the blender.
- Toss in a handful of ice cubes into the blender. This will help create a cold and refreshing smoothie.
- Secure the blender lid, and blend the ingredients until smooth and well combined. This usually takes a minute or two, depending on the power of your blender.
- If the smoothie is too thick, you can add more water or almond milk in small increments until you reach your desired consistency.
- Pour the smoothie into a glass and enjoy immediately.
- Optionally, you can garnish the smoothie with a sprinkle of cinnamon or a few carrot shreds for presentation.
- Feel free to customize the smoothie to your liking by adding ingredients like a scoop of protein powder, a tablespoon of chia seeds, or a drizzle of honey for sweetness.

Pineapple Mint Smoothie:

Ingredients:
- 1/2 cup pineapple chunks
- 1/4 cup fresh mint leaves

- 1/2 cucumber, peeled
- 1 cup coconut water
- Ice cubes

Instructions:
- Peel and chop the cucumber.
- Measure 1/2 cup of pineapple chunks.
- Pick and wash 1/4 cup of fresh mint leaves.
- Place the pineapple chunks, fresh mint leaves, and peeled cucumber in a blender.
- Pour 1 cup of coconut water into the blender.
- Add a handful of ice cubes to the blender. This will help make the smoothie cold and refreshing.
- Secure the blender lid, and blend all the ingredients until smooth. Depending on your blender, this may take 1-2 minutes.
- If the smoothie is too thick, you can add more coconut water and blend again until you reach your desired consistency.
- Taste the smoothie and adjust the sweetness or thickness by adding more pineapple, mint, or coconut water if needed.
- Pour the smoothie into glasses and serve immediately.
- Garnish the smoothie with a mint sprig or a slice of pineapple for an extra touch, (optional).
- Sip and enjoy your refreshing Pineapple Mint Smoothie!

Strawberry Kiwi Refresher

Ingredients:
- 1/2 cup strawberries, hulled and sliced
- 1 kiwi, peeled and sliced
- 1/2 cup unsweetened Greek yogurt
- 1 cup water
- Ice cubes

Instructions:
- Hull and slice the strawberries.
- Peel and slice the kiwi.
- Place the sliced strawberries and kiwi in a blender.
- Add 1/2 cup of unsweetened Greek yogurt to the blender.
- Measure 1 cup of water and pour it into the blender.
- Secure the blender lid and blend the ingredients until you achieve a smooth and creamy consistency.

- If the mixture is too thick, you can add more water in small increments and blend again until you reach the desired consistency.
- Add ice cubes to the blender for a refreshing and chilled drink.
- Blend once more to incorporate the ice cubes and make the refresher nice and cold.
- Pour the Strawberry Kiwi Refresher into glasses.
- Garnish with additional strawberry slices or kiwi pieces if desired.
- Serve immediately and enjoy your delicious and healthy Strawberry Kiwi Refresher!

Almond Joy Smoothie

Ingredients:
- 1/2 cup unsweetened coconut flakes
- 1 tablespoon almond butter
- 1/2 banana
- 1 cup unsweetened almond milk
- Ice cubes

Instructions:
- Measure 1/2 cup of unsweetened coconut flakes.
- Measure 1 tablespoon of almond butter.
- Peel and slice 1/2 banana.
- In a blender, add the unsweetened coconut flakes, almond butter, sliced banana, and 1 cup of unsweetened almond milk.
- Toss in a handful of ice cubes to the blender. The amount of ice can be adjusted based on your preference for thickness and coldness.
- Tighten the blender lid and blend the ingredients until smooth. This usually takes about 1-2 minutes, depending on the power of your blender.
- If the smoothie is too thick, you can add more almond milk in small increments and blend again until you reach the desired consistency.
- Taste the smoothie and adjust the sweetness or thickness if necessary. You can add a little honey or a sweetener of your choice if you prefer a sweeter taste.
- Pour the Almond Joy Smoothie into a glass.
- Optionally, you can garnish the smoothie with a sprinkle of coconut flakes or a drizzle of almond butter on top.
- Sip and enjoy your refreshing Almond Joy Smoothie!

Spinach and Pineapple Smoothie

Ingredients:
- 1 cup spinach leaves
- 1/2 cup pineapple chunks
- 1/2 banana

- 1 cup water or coconut water

Instructions:
- Gather all the ingredients.
- Place 1 cup of spinach leaves in the blender.
- Add 1/2 cup of pineapple chunks to the blender.
- Peel and add 1/2 banana to the other ingredients.
- Pour 1 cup of water or coconut water into the blender.
- Blend the ingredients until well combined and the smoothie reaches your desired consistency.
- Pour the smoothie into a glass and enjoy!

Raspberry Almond Protein Smoothie

Ingredients:
- 1/2 cup fresh or frozen raspberries
- 1 tablespoon almond butter
- 1 scoop vanilla protein powder
- 1 cup unsweetened almond milk
- Ice cubes (as desired)

Instructions:
- Measure out 1/2 cup of raspberries.
- Add 1 tablespoon of almond butter to the ingredients.
- Take 1 scoop of vanilla protein powder.
- Pour in 1 cup of unsweetened almond milk.
- Gather ice cubes as desired.
- In a blender, add the raspberries, almond butter, vanilla protein powder, and unsweetened almond milk.
- Toss in ice cubes according to your preference. Ice cubes will add a refreshing and chilled quality to the smoothie.
- Secure the blender lid and blend the ingredients until you achieve a smooth and creamy consistency. This usually takes about 1-2 minutes, depending on the power of your blender.
- Pause and check the consistency of the smoothie. If it's too thick, you can add more almond milk. If it's too thin, you can add a few more ice cubes or a bit of extra almond butter.
- Once the smoothie reaches the desired consistency, pour it into a glass.
- Optionally, you can garnish the smoothie with a few whole raspberries or a sprinkle of crushed almonds for added texture and visual appeal.
- Sip and enjoy your delicious Raspberry Almond Protein Smoothie!

Mango Ginger Zinger

Ingredients:
- 1/2 cup mango chunks
- 1/2 teaspoon grated ginger
- 1/2 cup Greek yogurt (unsweetened)
- 1 cup water
- Ice cubes

Instructions:
- Place 1/2 cup of mango chunks into a blender.
- Add 1/2 teaspoon of grated ginger to the blender.
- Measure and add 1/2 cup of unsweetened Greek yogurt to the blender.
- Pour 1 cup of water into the blender.
- Add ice cubes to the blender for a refreshing chill.
- Blend all the ingredients until smooth.
- Pour the Mango Ginger Zinger into a glass and enjoy your nutritious and flavorful drink!

Blueberry Walnut Smoothie

Ingredients:
- 1/2 cup blueberries
- 1 tablespoon chopped walnuts
- 1/2 cup spinach leaves
- 1 cup water or unsweetened almond milk

Instructions:
- Measure 1/2 cup of blueberries.
- Chop 1 tablespoon of walnuts.
- Add 1/2 cup of spinach leaves to the blender.
- Place the measured blueberries and chopped walnuts in the blender.
- Pour 1 cup of water or unsweetened almond milk into the blender.
- Blend the ingredients until well combined.
- Pour the smoothie into a glass and enjoy!

Chocolate Avocado Dream

Ingredients:
- 1/2 ripe avocado
- 1 tablespoon unsweetened cocoa powder
- 1/2 banana
- 1 cup unsweetened soy milk

- Ice cubes

Instructions:

- Prepare Ingredients: Ensure that the avocado is ripe and scoop out half of it. Peel and slice the banana.
- Combine Ingredients: In a blender, add the ripe avocado, unsweetened cocoa powder, sliced banana, and unsweetened soy milk.
- Add Ice Cubes: Toss in a handful of ice cubes. The amount of ice cubes can vary based on personal preference. They help make the drink cold and refreshing.
- Blend Until Creamy: Secure the blender lid and blend the ingredients until smooth and creamy. Make sure there are no avocado chunks left.
- Adjust Consistency: If the smoothie is too thick, you can add more soy milk in small increments until it reaches your desired consistency.
- Taste and Adjust: Taste the mixture and adjust the sweetness if needed. You can add a sweetener of your choice, such as honey or maple syrup, if the natural sweetness of the banana is not sufficient.
- Serve: Once the desired consistency and taste are achieved, pour the Chocolate Avocado Dream into a glass and enjoy!

Cranberry Orange Delight

Ingredients:

- 1/2 cup cranberries (fresh or frozen)
- 1/2 orange, peeled
- 1/2 cup Greek yogurt (unsweetened)
- 1 cup water
- Ice cubes

Instructions:

- If using fresh cranberries, wash them thoroughly. If using frozen cranberries, allow them to thaw slightly.
- Peel half of an orange.
- Place the cranberries, peeled orange, Greek yogurt, and water in a blender.
- Blend the ingredients until you achieve a smooth consistency. This may take a minute or two, depending on the power of your blender.
- If the mixture is too thick, you can add more water in small increments until you reach your desired consistency.
- Once the mixture is smooth and well-blended, add ice cubes to the blender. Blend again until the ice is crushed and the drink has a refreshing, chilled texture.
- Pour the Cranberry Orange Delight into glasses and serve immediately.

Peachy Keen Protein Smoothie

Ingredients:
- 1/2 cup sliced peaches
- 1 scoop vanilla protein powder
- 1/2 cup spinach leaves
- 1 cup water or unsweetened almond milk

Instructions:
- Wash and slice 1/2 cup of fresh peaches.
- Measure 1 scoop of vanilla protein powder.
- Measure 1/2 cup of spinach leaves.
- Place the sliced peaches, vanilla protein powder, and spinach leaves into a blender.
- Pour 1 cup of water or unsweetened almond milk into the blender.
- Blend the ingredients on high speed until the mixture is smooth and well combined.
- If the smoothie is too thick, you can add more water or almond milk in small increments until you reach your desired consistency.
- Pour the Peachy Keen Protein Smoothie into a glass.
- Garnish with additional peach slices or a sprinkle of protein powder if desired, and enjoy your nutritious and delicious smoothie!

Coconut Berry Bliss

Ingredients:
- 1/2 cup mixed berries (strawberries, blueberries)
- 1/2 cup coconut milk (unsweetened)
- 1/2 banana
- 1 tablespoon chia seeds
- Ice cubes

Instructions:
- Wash the mixed berries thoroughly.
- Peel and slice the banana.
- In a blender, add the mixed berries, sliced banana, and chia seeds.
- Pour in 1/2 cup of unsweetened coconut milk.
- Toss in a handful of ice cubes. The amount can vary depending on your preference for thickness and chilliness.
- Blend all the ingredients together until you achieve a smooth consistency. This usually takes a few minutes.
- If the smoothie is too thick, you can add more coconut milk or a bit of water and blend again until you reach your desired consistency.
- Pour the blended mixture into a glass or a bowl.

- You can garnish with additional berries, chia seeds, or a slice of banana on top if you'd like.
- Your Coconut Berry Bliss is ready to be enjoyed! This smoothie is not only delicious but also packed with nutrients from the berries, banana, and chia seeds.

Bonus Recipes

Blueberry Almond Chia Pudding

Ingredients
- 1/2 cup chia seeds
- 1 cup unsweetened almond milk (or other plant-based milk)
- 1/4 cup fresh or frozen blueberries
- 1 tablespoon honey or maple syrup (optional)
- 1/2 teaspoon vanilla extract
- 1/4 cup toasted slivered almonds

Instructions.
- The blueberries, almond milk, chia seeds, vanilla extract, honey (if used), and maple syrup should all be combined in a jar or dish.
- Allow the mixture to settle for 5 minutes so the chia seeds can absorb part of the liquid.
- Refrigerate the dish or container for at least 2 hours, or overnight.
- When preparing to serve, thoroughly stir the pudding. If desired, top with toasted almonds and extra blueberries.

Tips
- Use less almond milk for a thicker pudding. Use extra almond milk to make a thinner pudding.
- In this recipe, you may use whatever sort of milk you choose.
- You may use another sweetener, such agave nectar or stevia, if you don't have honey or maple syrup.
- The pudding may be stored in the refrigerator for up to three days.

Variations.
- For added flavor, add a sprinkle of cinnamon or nutmeg to the pudding.
- For extra protein, add a teaspoon of almond butter or peanut butter.
- Fresh fruit, such as strawberries, bananas, or peaches, may be sprinkled on top of the pudding.
- Instead of almonds, use a different nut, such as chopped walnuts or pecans.
- I hope you love this recipe!

Apple Cinnamon Chia Pudding

Ingredients:
- 1/4 cup chia seeds
- 1 cup unsweetened almond milk (or other plant-based milk)
- 1/2 cup unsweetened applesauce

- 1/2 teaspoon ground cinnamon
- 1/4 teaspoon vanilla extract
- 1/4 cup chopped apple (optional)
- 1 tablespoon chopped nuts or seeds (optional)

Instructions:
- Mix the applesauce, almond milk, chia seeds, cinnamon, and vanilla essence in a bowl.
- To make sure the chia seeds are spread equally, let the mixture settle for five minutes before whisking it once more.
- The dish should be covered and chilled for at least four hours, or perhaps overnight.
- Spoon pudding into dishes and serve immediately. Add diced apple and, if like, nuts or seeds on top.

Tips:
- Add a spoonful of honey or maple syrup for a sweeter pudding.
- Pumpkin puree or mashed bananas may be used in place of applesauce if you don't have any.
- Additional toppings for your pudding include granola, berries, or coconut flakes.

Avocado Toast With Egg, Arugula And Bacon

Ingredients:
1 slice of hearty bread (sourdough, whole wheat, or rye work well)
- 1/2 small avocado, mashed
- Pinch of salt and pepper
- 1/2 cup arugula
- 1 slice bacon
- 1/2 teaspoon extra-virgin olive oil
- 1 large egg

Instructions:
- Toast the bread: Place the bread slice in a toaster or under a broiler until golden brown.
- Prepare the avocado: While the bread is toasting, mash the avocado half with a fork and season it with salt and pepper.
- Assemble the base: Spread the mashed avocado onto the toasted bread.
- Add the arugula: Top the avocado with a layer of peppery arugula.
- Cook the bacon: Cook the bacon slice in a skillet over medium heat until crisp. Drain the excess fat on a paper towel-lined plate.

- Cook the egg: Heat the olive oil in the same skillet over medium heat. Crack the egg into the pan and cook it to your desired doneness. A sunny-side up egg is classic for this recipe, but you can also cook it over easy or scrambled.
- Assemble the toast: Top the avocado toast with the cooked egg and crumble the bacon over it.

Tips:
- For an extra burst of flavor, drizzle the finished toast with a squeeze of lemon juice or balsamic vinegar.
- If you don't have arugula, you can substitute baby spinach or another leafy green.
- To make this a vegetarian dish, simply omit the bacon.
- This recipe is easily customizable! Feel free to add other toppings like sliced tomato, red onion, or crumbled cheese.

Avocado Egg-Toast

Ingredients
- 1 slice of bread (sourdough, whole wheat, or your favorite kind)
- 1/4 of a ripe avocado
- 1 large egg
- Salt and pepper to taste
- Optional toppings: red pepper flakes, hot sauce, Everything Bagel Seasoning, crumbled feta cheese, chopped tomatoes, and microgreens

Instructions:
- Toast the bread to your desired doneness.
- While the bread is toasting, mash the avocado with a fork in a small bowl. Season with salt and pepper to taste.
- Cook the egg however you like: fried, scrambled, poached, or boiled.
- Spread the mashed avocado on the toast.
- Top with the cooked egg.
- Add any of your desired toppings.

Tips;
- Use ripe avocados that are soft to the touch but not mushy.
- Toast your bread to a nice golden brown so it can hold up to the toppings.
- Don't overcook the egg. You want the yolk to be runny or soft-cooked.
- Get creative with your toppings! There are endless possibilities.
- I hope you enjoy this delicious and easy recipe!

Variations;

- Spicy Avocado Egg Toast: Add a pinch of red pepper flakes or a drizzle of hot sauce to the mashed avocado.
- Mediterranean Avocado Egg Toast: Top with crumbled feta cheese, chopped tomatoes, and a drizzle of olive oil.
- Everything Bagel Avocado Egg Toast: Sprinkle Everything Bagel Seasoning on the toast before adding the avocado and egg.
- Smoked Salmon Avocado Egg Toast: Top with smoked salmon, cream cheese, and dill.
- No matter how you make it, avocado egg toast is a surefire way to start your day off right.

Peanut Butter And Apple Toast

Ingredients:

- 1 slice of bread (your choice! Whole wheat, sourdough, rye, or even a bagel work great)
- 1-2 tablespoons peanut butter (creamy or crunchy, depending on your preference)
- 1/4 apple, thinly sliced (any variety works, but sweeter apples like Honeycrisp or Fuji are particularly good)
- Optional toppings: cinnamon, honey, maple syrup, chopped nuts, chia seeds, dried fruit, etc.

Instructions:

- Toast your bread to your desired level of doneness.
- Spread the peanut butter over the toast.
- Arrange the apple slices on top of the peanut butter.
- Sprinkle with your desired toppings (if using).
- Enjoy immediately!

Tips:

- For a warm treat, microwave the apple slices for 30-60 seconds before topping the toast.
- If you're using crunchy peanut butter, be sure to spread it evenly to avoid clumps.
- Drizzle with a little honey or maple syrup for extra sweetness.
- Get creative with your toppings! Try chopped nuts, chia seeds, dried fruit, or even a sprinkle of granola.
- This recipe is easily doubled or tripled to feed a crowd.

Avocado Egg Salad Sandwiches

Ingredients:

For the egg salad:

- 1 ripe avocado, peeled and pitted
- 3 hard-boiled eggs, peeled and chopped

- 1/4 cup finely chopped red onion
- 2 tablespoons chopped fresh parsley
- 1 tablespoon chopped fresh chives
- 1 tablespoon lemon juice
- 2 tablespoons plain Greek yogurt or mayonnaise
- Salt and freshly ground black pepper, to taste

For the sandwiches:
- 4 slices whole-wheat bread, toasted
- 2 leaves romaine lettuce

Instructions:
- Make the egg salad: Mash the avocado in a medium bowl with a fork until mostly smooth.
- Stir in the chopped eggs, red onion, parsley, chives, lemon juice, Greek yogurt or mayonnaise, salt, and pepper until well combined.
- Assemble the sandwiches: Spread the egg salad on the toasted bread slices. Top each with a romaine lettuce leaf and another slice of bread.
- Enjoy! Serve the sandwiches immediately.

Tips:
- For a spicier egg salad, add a finely chopped jalapeño pepper to the mixture.
- If you don't have romaine lettuce, you can use any other type of lettuce or even spinach.
- You can also use this egg salad recipe to fill wraps or pita bread.
- If you have leftover egg salad, store it in an airtight container in the refrigerator for up to 2 days.

Strawberry Kiwi Cheesecake Toast

Ingredients:
- 2 slices thick-cut bread (brioche, challah, or French bread work well)
- 2 tablespoons cream cheese, softened
- 1 tablespoon powdered sugar
- 1/4 teaspoon vanilla extract
- 1/4 cup fresh strawberries, sliced
- 1/4 cup fresh kiwi, sliced
- Honey, for drizzling (optional)
- Mint leaves, for garnish (optional)

Instructions:
- Toast the bread to your desired doneness.
- In a small bowl, mix together the cream cheese, powdered sugar, and vanilla extract until smooth.
- Spread the cream cheese mixture evenly on one slice of toast.
- Top the cream cheese with the sliced strawberries and kiwi.
- Drizzle with honey, if desired.
- Garnish with mint leaves, if desired.
- Serve immediately and enjoy!

Tips:
- For a richer flavor, you can toast the bread in butter or olive oil.
- If you don't have fresh strawberries or kiwi, you can use frozen fruit that has been thawed.
- You can also add other toppings to your toast, such as granola, chopped nuts, or whipped cream.
- I hope you enjoy this recipe!

Variations you can try
- Mascarpone Cheesecake Toast: Use mascarpone cheese instead of cream cheese for a lighter and tangier flavor.
- Blueberry Kiwi Cheesecake Toast: Use blueberries instead of strawberries for a different flavor combination.
- Chocolate Hazelnut Cheesecake Toast: Spread Nutella on the toast before adding the cream cheese mixture.
- Deconstructed Cheesecake Toast: Crumble graham crackers on top of the toast before adding the cream cheese mixture.

Southwestern Waffle

Ingredients:
- 2 eggs, separated
- 1 ¾ cups warm milk
- ⅓ cup butter, melted
- 2 tablespoons honey
- 1 ¼ cups cornmeal
- 1 cup all-purpose flour
- 4 teaspoons baking powder
- 2 teaspoons salt
- ½ cup corn
- 2 green chile peppers, seeded and minced (more or less to taste)

- Vegetable oil, for greasing the waffle iron

Instructions:
- Preheat your waffle maker based on the instructions on the packet.
- Beat the egg whites in a large bowl until firm peaks form.
- Whisk the egg yolks, milk, melted butter, and honey in a another basin.
- Mix the flour, baking powder, cornmeal, and salt in a separate basin.
- Add the corn and green chili peppers after carefully combining the dry and wet ingredients.
- Apply vegetable oil to your waffle iron to grease it.
- Transfer around ½ cup of batter onto the waffle iron and let it cook for 3–4 minutes, or until it becomes crispy and golden brown.
- Proceed with the leftover batter.
- With your preferred toppings, such avocado, black beans, salsa, sour cream, or cheese, serve your waffles hot.

Tips:
- Add a little sprinkle of cayenne pepper to the batter for a hotter waffle.
- Red bell peppers or poblano peppers may be used in place of green chile peppers.
- Instead of using milk in this recipe, you may use buttermilk.
- Preheat your oven to 200°F (93°C). While you prepare the remaining batter, lay the waffles on a baking sheet and keep them warm in the oven.

Spring Green Frittata

Ingredients;
- 1 tablespoon olive oil
- 1 medium onion, thinly sliced
- 2 cloves garlic, minced
- 8 ounces Swiss chard, roughly chopped (or arugula or Asian greens)
- 6 ounces button mushrooms, sliced
- 4 ounces feta cheese, crumbled
- 12 large eggs
- 1/2 cup milk (or unsweetened almond milk for a vegan option)
- 1/4 teaspoon salt
- Freshly ground black pepper
- 1/4 cup chopped fresh herbs (such as chives, parsley, or dill)

Instructions:

- Preheat oven to 375°F (190°C). Heat olive oil in a large ovenproof skillet over medium heat. Add onion and cook until softened, about 5 minutes. Add garlic and cook for 30 seconds more.
- Stir in Swiss chard (or arugula or Asian greens) and mushrooms. Cook until greens are wilted and mushrooms are softened, about 5 minutes. Drain any excess liquid.
- Sprinkle feta cheese over the vegetables.
- In a large bowl, whisk together eggs, milk, salt, and pepper. Pour egg mixture over the vegetables and cheese in the skillet.
- Transfer the skillet to the oven and bake for 20-25 minutes, or until the frittata is set and golden brown around the edges.
- Garnish with chopped fresh herbs and serve immediately.

Tips:

- For a richer flavor, use goat cheese instead of feta.
- To make the frittata ahead of time, let it cool completely, then store it in the refrigerator for up to 3 days. Reheat gently in a skillet over low heat or in the oven at 325°F (165°C) until warmed through.
- Serve the frittata with a side of crusty bread or a simple salad.

Tomato And Olive Dinner Frittata

Ingredients:
- 1 tablespoon olive oil
- 1/2 onion, chopped
- 2 cloves garlic, minced
- 1/2 red bell pepper, chopped
- 1/2 green bell pepper, chopped
- 1/4 cup sun-dried tomatoes, chopped
- 1/2 cup kalamata olives, pitted and halved
- 6 large eggs
- 1/4 cup milk
- 1/2 cup grated Parmesan cheese
- 1/4 teaspoon dried oregano
- Salt and pepper to taste
- Fresh basil, for garnish (optional)

Instructions:

- Preheat the oven to 400°F (200°C). Heat olive oil in a 10-inch ovenproof skillet over medium heat.
- Add the onion and cook until softened, about 5 minutes. Add garlic, bell peppers, and sun-dried tomatoes, and cook until softened, about 5 minutes more.
- Stir in olives and cook for 1 minute. In a large bowl, whisk together eggs, milk, Parmesan cheese, oregano, salt, and pepper. Pour the egg mixture into the skillet over the vegetables, and cook until the edges begin to set, about 5 minutes.
- Transfer the skillet to the oven and bake for 10-15 minutes, or until the eggs are set and the top is golden brown. Garnish with fresh basil, if desired.

Tips:

- For a vegetarian frittata, omit the bacon.
- You can use any type of olives you like.
- Serve the frittata with a side of crusty bread or salad.
- Here are some additional notes about the recipe:

Additional Notes About The Recipe:

- This recipe is easy to adapt to your dietary needs. For example, you can use low-fat or fat-free milk, skip the cheese, or use a different type of cheese.
- You can also add other vegetables to the frittata, such as spinach, mushrooms, or zucchini.
- If you don't have an ovenproof skillet, you can transfer the frittata to a baking dish after cooking the vegetables.

www.ingramcontent.com/pod-product-compliance
Lightning Source LLC
Chambersburg PA
CBHW080927260726
48661CB00010B/3836